PICTURE THE POSSIBILITIES WITH

A FLAT STOMACH ASAP.

Do for yourself what these people have done:

- ### LOST 25³/₄ POUNDS OF FAT

"My clothes size dropped from a 16 to a 5-to-7. It's so much fun shopping now because I can try selections from the junior department."

—Paige Arnold, age 27

- ### TRIMMED 10³/₄ INCHES OFF WAIST

"It's depressing to be kidded about being pregnant—especially if you're a man. Now my pot belly is gone, thanks to Dr. Darden's outstanding program."

—Ken Howell, age 59

- ### ADDED CURVES IN THE RIGHT PLACES

"I gained 40 pounds during my last pregnancy and much of this weight was hanging around a year later. The ASAP plan really focused on reshaping my stomach and rebuilding my thighs and arms. As a result, I look years younger."

—Karen Purdy, age 29

- ### REMOVED 71¹/₄ POUNDS OF FAT

"I was a skillful athlete in high school and college, but I always was self-conscious about taking off my shirt. My flabby belly was embarrassing. Today, my stomach is hard, my body is lean, and I feel great about both."

—Barry Ozer, age 25

- ### SUPPORTED JOINT PARTICIPATION

"It was a terrific experience for both of us. We planned, shopped, cooked, ate, and worked out together. Best of all, we succeeded together."

—Tammy and Joe Gentry, ages 35 and 36

Before-and-after photos of these and
many other success stories appear throughout

A FLAT STOMACH ASAP.

Other Books by Ellington Darden, Ph.D.

32 Days to a 32-Inch Waist
Two Weeks to a Tighter Tummy
Nutrition for Athletes
The Nautilus Book
The Nautilus Bodybuilding Book
The Nautilus Diet
High-Intensity Strength Training
New High-Intensity Bodybuilding
The Athlete's Guide to Sports Medicine
The Six-Week Fat-to-Muscle Makeover
The Complete Encyclopedia of Weight Loss, Body Shaping,
    and Slenderizing
High-Intensity Home Training
Soft Steps to a Hard Body
Body Defining
Living Longer Stronger

A FLAT STOMACH
ASAP™

the **Breakthrough Plan**
for the **Look You Want**
in **Just Six Weeks**

Ellington Darden, Ph.D.

POCKET BOOKS
New York   London   Toronto   Sydney

The author is not a physician and this book is not intended as a substitute for the medical advice of a physician. Before beginning this, or any other weight-loss program, the reader should get a medical checkup and consult with a physician in regard to matters relating to the reader's health and in particular to the weight-loss program the reader intends to follow, as well as consulting about any symptoms that may require diagnosis or medical attention. The author and publisher disclaim any liability arising directly or indirectly from the use of this book.

An *Original* Publication of POCKET BOOKS

POCKET BOOKS, a division of Simon & Schuster Inc.
1230 Avenue of the Americas, New York, NY 10020

Library of Congress Cataloging-in-Publication Data

Darden, Ellington, 1943–
    A flat stomach ASAP : the breakthrough plan for the look you want
in just six weeks / Ellington Darden.
        p.   cm.
    ISBN-13: 978-0-671-01408-7
    ISBN-10:   0-671-01408-0
    1. Weight loss.   2. Abdomen—Muscles.   3. Exercise.   4. Reducing
diets.   I. Title.
RM222.2.D2894   1998
613.7—dc21   97-31233
                                                                  CIP

First Pocket Books trade paperback printing January 1998

20 19 18 17

Cover design by Lisa Litwack
Cover photo courtesy of Tony Stone Images
Cover inset photo courtesy of Superstock

Printed in the U.S.A.

ACKNOWLEDGMENTS

Sincere thanks go to the following people who helped in the preparation of *A Flat Stomach ASAP:*

Stedman Mays read the proposal and initial draft and offered a number of valuable suggestions.

Kathy Pishotta input the manuscript into her word processor and made the necessary revisions.

Emily Bestler and Leslie Stern edited the book.

Timothy Tew produced the exercise photographs.

Ken Hutchins took the before-and-after pictures.

Tom Hall scanned many of the book's photographs.

Lydia Maree and Josh Miller contributed to the exercise training.

David Hudlow, Michael Spillane, and Karen Coley-Cannon helped with the measurements.

Paige Arnold, Jeffrey Arnold, Ana Rocha, Stacey Ferrari, Kerry Hamilton, Lisa Danver, Barry Ozer, Mike Derringer, and Craig Wilburn—all of whom went through the program—demonstrated the recommended exercises.

Tim Patterson supported the entire project with skill and guidance.

Special appreciation goes to Joe Cirulli and the Gainesville Health & Fitness Center and to all the women and men who participated in the research for this book.

CONTENTS

PART THREE

APPLICATION

PART FOUR

PERSISTENCE

Introduction:
Straight Talk About Stomach Flattening

What body parts do people most want to improve? NordicTrack recently commissioned a survey to find out.

Abdominals captured first place with 60 percent of the vote. *Legs* finished a distant second with 14 percent.

Men and women were identical in their preferences. Both wanted exercise equipment and expert instruction on how to get flat, hard, muscular stomachs.

These findings and similar ones opened the door wide for home abdominal machines. And infomercial television marketers rushed to meet this need.

Important: If you're one of the six million people who purchased a home abdominal machine in 1996 and 1997, you may have been persuaded to buy for the wrong reason.

Perhaps you were influenced to think that doing a few sit-up exercises a day will burn midsection fat and define your waist? In a matter of weeks, if you believe some of the advertisements, you'll develop either a flat sexy stomach or rock-hard abs.

These claims and subsequent beliefs are *false*.

People with protruding bellies have excessive fat around their midsections. Contracting the underlying muscles will help—but real progress will be made only when body-fat levels are significantly reduced. Reducing fat efficiently requires *dieting*.

"But wait a minute," you might be saying, "I thought all this could be done without dieting? That's why I bought the abdominal machine."

Sorry to disappoint you, but the answer is *no*.

Sure, exercise burns calories, and calories can come from your fatty deposits. The problem is that exercise for your midsection melts away few calories.

Abdominal exercises, by the best calculations, require an average of 7.5 calories per minute. Thus, each of those highly advertised five-minute workouts uses 37.5 calories. It would take seven hours and forty-seven minutes of continuous repetitions, or ninety-three days of five-minute workouts, to get rid of 3,500 calories or one pound of fat.

From these numbers you should recognize how inefficient abdominal exercise is in the fat-loss process.

Exercise is only a moderate calorie burner. But even so, it is absolutely essential for maximum fat loss.

Why? Because strength training, the type of exercise utilized in this book, stimulates your muscles to grow larger and stronger. Stronger muscles speed up your metabolism so you require more calories each day.

Muscle, not exercise, is your foremost calorie burner.

The key to building stronger muscles is to eliminate most of the momentum from the strength training. Doing so demands that all movements be performed slowly and smoothly. This book illustrates how to do each of the recommended exercises slowly and smoothly in perfect form.

What Is ASAP?

ASAP denotes more than *as soon as possible.*

A stands for *Awareness*—how to understand and evaluate your midsection fatness and fitness.

S stands for *Science*—how to rely on solid facts, not popular fictions, to change the shape and condition of your body.

A stands for *Application*—how to combine research and facts into a result-producing program.

P stands for *Persistence*—how to sustain the course, reach your goal, and maintain a lean middle permanently.

The book is also organized into four parts: Awareness, Science, Application, and Persistence. To further reinforce the acronym, all chapter titles under each part begin with the same first letter.

A Flat Stomach ASAP is designed specifically for men and women who are pressed for time. It's for busy people who are always on the move. It's for people who respond well to a plan, a daily and weekly course of action.

With proper awareness, science, application, and persistence, almost anyone can get a lean midsection *as soon as possible.*

Diet has often been called a four-letter word that brings to mind calorie counting, tasteless foods, and hunger pangs. By applying new discoveries in food technology, dieting doesn't have to be a bad experience. If you accept a reduced-calorie eating plan for what it is—a necessary step in the fat-loss process—you can adapt your lifestyle to cope with the discipline that is required to be successful. This course incorporates the best dieting guidelines that science has to offer.

Superhydration, the sipping of large amounts of ice-cold water each day, is one of the most important of those guidelines. Superhydration synergizes your eating and exercising. It accelerates stomach flattening.

You'll learn all about superhydration, diet, exercise, and much more in *A Flat Stomach ASAP*.

Best of all, the title *A Flat Stomach ASAP*, even though it contains a provocative acronym, is no gimmick. It can happen to you!

But let me give you the straight talk. Losing pounds and inches of fat from your waist requires discipline. The entire process demands *hard work*.

Have you ever accomplished anything meaningful in your life that didn't demand focus and discipline? Probably not.

I find that people accept hard work—if—they see results *fast*.

With *A Flat Stomach ASAP*, many individuals lose 7 to 11 pounds of fat and 2½ inches off their midsections in the first two weeks.

Continuing the program for six weeks, the average man can expect to drop 23 pounds of fat and 4 inches off his belly. A typical woman can expect to shed 15 pounds of fat and 3½ inches off her middle.

Achieving a lean body and a flat stomach has never been easier.

Get ready to lose maximum pounds and inches quickly.

Get ready to understand and apply *A Flat Stomach ASAP*.

AWARENESS

Part One

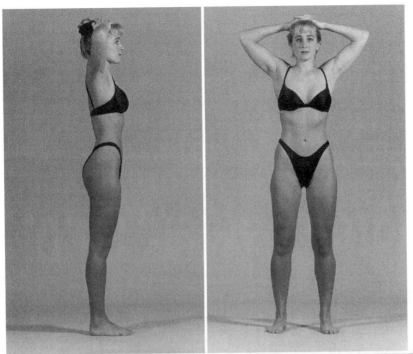
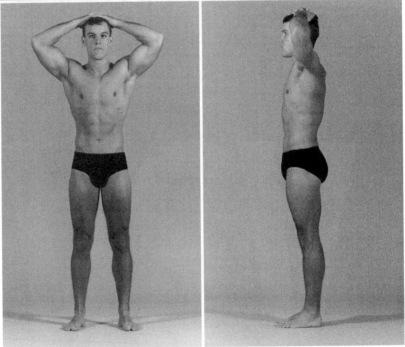

The midsections of Jenny Rogers and Mike Derringer are excellent examples of flat stomachs. Jenny and Mike had just completed two weeks of the ASAP course. Jenny lost 7½ pounds of fat and Mike dropped 12 pounds. Notice the contours and lines that they have on the front and sides of their midsections.

1

ANSWER:
SOLVE YOUR BULGING BELLY

"ABS-olutely fabulous: The craving for chiseled stomach muscles," blazed the front-page headline in *USA Today* (May 21, 1996). Placed throughout this article were pictures of the rippling midsections of Sylvester Stallone, Jackie Joyner-Kersee, Janet Jackson, and a Calvin Klein underwear model.

"It used to be enough just to be thin," wrote Joe Urshel, the author of this cover story. "No more. Now you must have great abs."

Understanding the Obsession

Why are Americans so obsessed with flat stomachs and muscular waists?

Much of this obsession has to do with the law of supply and demand. What is scarce and difficult to achieve is valuable—not only valuable but attractive.

Twenty years ago, according to Ann Scott Beller, Americans were the third fattest people in the world—ranking behind the Russians and Germans. Not so today. In 1995, we were elevated to the number one position.

As if this number one position isn't secure enough, we're trying to run up the score.

A study released by the Harris poll in February of 1996 shows that 74 percent of Americans twenty-five years of age and older are overweight. Similar Harris surveys found that 58 percent were overweight in 1983, 64 percent in 1990, 69 percent in 1994, and 71 percent in 1995.

If this rate of increase—approximately 1.1 percent per year—continues unabated, then by the year 2021 every adult in the United States over twenty-five will be overweight.

Obviously, we're becoming more and more obsessed with flat stomachs, great abdominals, and leanness in general—because we're seeing fewer and fewer of what we find attractive. Remember the law of supply and demand? It applies not only to economics but also to body parts.

The opposite of a flat stomach is a protruding or bulging belly. The opposite of leanness is fatness.

Research reveals a direct relationship between flat and lean, and between protrusion and fatness. A person with a protruding belly has too much overall body fat.

Thus, one important step in getting a flat stomach is to reduce overall fat. Other than surgery, which I don't recommend, there's no way to remove *only* belly fat. But most people do have the genetics to lose the majority of fat from their thickest storage spots, which is often the stomach area.

Before getting into the cure or answer for a bulging belly, it's important to understand briefly some of the causes.

Why Americans Are Getting Fatter

Here are the primary reasons why Americans are gaining fat pounds and inches:

- The leisure-time activities of most people increasingly revolve around television, movies, and other passive activities. As a consequence, most adults lose one-half pound of muscle mass per year, which causes a one-half percent decline in metabolic rate.
- Even with all the media emphasis on the physical fitness boom in the last two decades, the end result has been a bust. Millions of people have been injured from exercise, and even more have received no results. Statistics show that fewer than 10 percent of adults do anything classified as vigorous at least three times per week.
- We've been blitzed by a complex array of eating advice involving such things as fat grams, antioxidants, sugar-free, junk meals, and health foods. Such advice hasn't worked. Although we are consuming more low-fat and sugar-free foods than we did a decade ago, we have compensated by eating more of almost everything else as well. As a result, most

adults add 1½ pounds of fat per year to their bodies and accumulate a large amount of this fat around their midsections.

- Research indicates that as most people age, they become drier. This drying occurs throughout the body: skin, hair, internal organs, bones, muscles, and even fatty tissues. Such dehydration can go unnoticed for years. Even mild dehydration accentuates the gradual loss of muscle and the gradual gain of fat.
- More bad and good information exists today than ever before concerning eating and exercising. Unfortunately, bad information—which is protected by our country's freedom of speech and freedom of the press—is increasing in disproportionately large amounts compared to good information.

The Answer to the Problem

Logically, the answer must involve corrections for all of the causes, and it does.

- *Loss of muscle mass:* Strength training rebuilds lost muscle mass. Strength training involves the use of dumbbells, barbells, lightweight home machines, heavy-duty health club equipment, or even movements using your own body weight.
- *Unsafe and unproductive exercise:* Any type of exercise can be unsafe and unproductive, at least from a muscle-building capacity, if it is performed in a fast, jerky fashion, or if it is repeated for longer than two minutes. The safest and most productive form of strength training is called super slow. Each repetition requires fifteen seconds and is repeated four to eight times.
- *Complex dietary guidelines that lead to the overconsumption of calories and the increase in body fat:* Simple, specific guidelines direct a person in exactly what to eat each meal. Five minimeals a day teach portion control, facilitate appetite regulation, and accelerate stomach flattening.
- *Dehydration:* The cure for dehydration involves more than gulping down a little extra water. It entails the systematic and progressive sipping of at least one gallon of ice-cold water each day. Superhydration is the name I've given this process. When superhydration is correctly combined with the strength training and minimeals, you get a compounding, synergistic effect: *you lose fat pounds and inches faster than ever!*
- *Too much misleading information concerning courses of action:* Having all parts

to the puzzle is important. But equally important is the way and order in which you put them together. Too many courses of action quickly become a part of the problem rather than a reliable solution. A carefully organized six-week program—with daily guidelines centering around eating, superhydrating, exercising, and resting—combats misinformation and yields fast fat loss.

Science: The Most Important Cornerstone

As stated in the introduction, *ASAP* is a common acronym for *as soon as possible.* These letters also stand for Awareness, Science, Application, and Persistence, which are the cornerstones of stomach flattening.

Science is the most important cornerstone.

At the heart of science is the tension between contradictory attitudes: an openness to new ideas, no matter how bizarre they may be, and a skeptical scrutiny of both new and old ideas. The battle between creative and skeptical thinking keeps science on track.

For more than twenty-five years I've been, in a sense, a scientist. Even before I began college, I had a curiosity about facts and a desire to search out the truth. For most of my fifty-three years I've had a strong interest in physical fitness.

I graduated from Florida State University in 1972 with a Ph.D. in exercise science and then completed two years of postdoctoral study in the food and nutrition department. I was director of research for Nautilus Sports/Medical Industries for seventeen years. As a result, I've read, studied, and reviewed much of the scientific literature on fitness. Furthermore, I've researched and published more than 350 articles and forty-four books on food, nutrition, fat loss, and strength training.

In the process, I've trained more than four thousand men and six thousand women on various eating and exercising plans. My overriding objective was always to find the most effective and efficient way to reduce fat and build muscle.

I can truthfully say that *A Flat Stomach ASAP* is the best fat-loss program that I've ever developed.

Some of the success of the ASAP program is connected to a popular home abdominal machine called the AB Trainer.

AB Trainer™ Connection

While I was director of research for Nautilus Sports/Medical Industries, I saw dozens of prototypes for new exercise machines that came mostly from amateur designers. Some of them were as big as an automobile and others were as small as a birdcage. Some came equipped with gears and motors, others with lights and beepers. Without exception, the pieces I examined were neither practical nor an improvement over what was already available.

So you might say I was a bit skeptical when I was approached by Don Brown, the owner of a large fitness center in Chester, New Jersey. I had just finished one of my presentations at a Nautilus Training Seminar in New York City during July of 1994, and Don was one of the attendees. Don invited me to his hotel room to try his new invention.

As I entered his room, I saw it: the AB Trainer. It was about the size of a small rocking chair with the back missing. One of Don's buddies was on the floor using it, smoothly crunching his abdominals into a tight muscular contraction.

Instantly, I recognized the potential for this device.

The AB Trainer was small, lightweight, easy to use, and safe. But more important, it forced you to do a trunk curl or abdominal crunch in the most productive manner.

I understood the AB Trainer, tried it, felt it in my middle, and told Don I'd be interested in doing some research with it.

Three months later, Don shipped me six AB Trainers for use in a specially designed stomach-flattening project. By mid-1995, after having put three groups of subjects through my scientific protocols, I had meaningful data to share.

Don Brown and I joined forces and developed "The 10-Day Quick-Start Program for a Flat Stomach," which features the AB Trainer. This course is packaged with each AB Trainer that is sold. Furthermore, it's a salient part of the 28-minute infomercial that was produced by Stilson & Stilson.

You may have seen me on the AB Trainer infomercial, which has been frequently shown on many cable television stations throughout most of 1996. Perhaps you've ordered one of the AB Trainer units or purchased one from a large department store in your city. More than one million of the machines were sold in 1996.

Even though Don Brown owns the original patent for an abdominal machine that supplies roller-frame support for the head and arms, his concept has been copied, renamed, manufactured, and sold by many companies. At last count, Don had filed lawsuits for patent violations against twelve different manufacturers.

I know the AB Trainer is a quality machine. I've tested and used it extensively with several hundred participants in my programs at the Gainesville Health & Fitness Center in Gainesville, Florida. I can't be sure of the other home abdominal machines. Some of them look like they might be well constructed and some of them appear flimsy.

But I'm sure of one thing: Whatever abdominal equipment you own or have access to, you'll get much better results if you use it according to the super-slow style and the ASAP approach that I describe in this book. The same advice goes to those of you who don't have access to any equipment. You can still get good

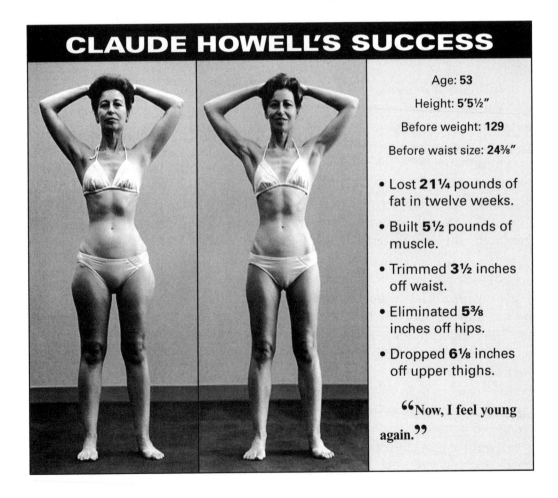

CLAUDE HOWELL'S SUCCESS

Age: **53**

Height: **5'5½"**

Before weight: **129**

Before waist size: **24⅜"**

- Lost **21¼** pounds of fat in twelve weeks.

- Built **5½** pounds of muscle.

- Trimmed **3½** inches off waist.

- Eliminated **5⅜** inches off hips.

- Dropped **6⅛** inches off upper thighs.

"Now, I feel young again."

results from using my ASAP approach to freehand exercise that involves your own body weight.

Success Stories with ASAP

The ASAP program has been tested, evaluated, improved, and retested on thousands of people—people of all ages, shapes, and sizes.

Success stories of some of these men and women—including before-and-after photographs—appear throughout this book. All of the comparison pictures are standardized and unretouched. Although each person has unique characteristics, each person's body also resembles other bodies in some respects. It will be useful for you to examine these photographs carefully for body shapes similar to your own. Doing so will help you get a realistic view of what you can achieve.

The first two success stories feature a married couple, Claude and Ken Howell.

Claude: "I Used to Have Such a Small Waist"

Claude Howell, fifty-three, is an office manager for an architectural firm. She had been fairly active for most of her life and remembered that her extra weight didn't start hanging on until she reached fifty. "Within a year or so," Claude recalls, "I had this pouch under my navel and these saddlebags around my hips and thighs."

"I used to have such a trim waist and slender hips in my twenties and thirties. I joined the program for one reason: I wanted my figure to look like it did twenty years ago."

Claude quickly turned into one of the most disciplined women that I've ever worked with. She progressed through two back-to-back six-week courses.

And it showed—big time.

Claude lost 21$\frac{1}{4}$ pounds of fat and trimmed 3$\frac{1}{2}$ inches off her waist, 5$\frac{3}{8}$ inches off her hips, and 6$\frac{1}{8}$ inches off her upper thighs. Equally important, she built 5$\frac{1}{2}$ pounds of muscle.

And get this, after twelve weeks her waistline measured an incredible 20$\frac{7}{8}$ inches. I've never, in more than thirty years of measuring adult waistlines, recorded a number that small.

Was Claude pleased? Afterward, here's what she told me.

"Last weekend, I visited my hometown. It was hot outside so I wore shorts and a halter top. I was talking with the elderly man across the street from where I grew up when suddenly his wife appeared. The first thing she said was she had to find out who that attractive teenage girl was her husband was flirting with. That teenage girl was me, and I'll be fifty-four years old next month.''

Ken: "Talk about a Classic Pot Belly"

Claude's success also got the attention of her husband, Ken Howell. At fifty-nine years of age, he's an engineer at Texas Instruments. "This incredible program," remembers Ken, "that's all I heard about for weeks—as I drank and snacked each night in front of the TV set. With this classic pot belly of mine, I didn't need much convincing to give it a try."

Once Ken started on the program, he displayed the same discipline and work ethic that Claude had applied so successfully.

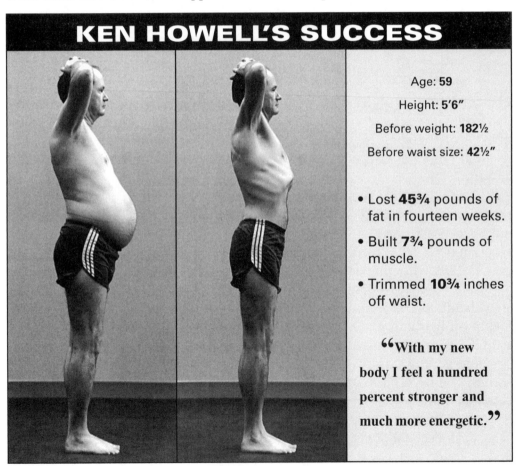

KEN HOWELL'S SUCCESS

Age: **59**

Height: **5'6"**

Before weight: **182½**

Before waist size: **42½"**

- Lost **45¾** pounds of fat in fourteen weeks.
- Built **7¾** pounds of muscle.
- Trimmed **10¾** inches off waist.

"With my new body I feel a hundred percent stronger and much more energetic."

Three months later, Ken looked like a different man. He shed 45¾ pounds of fat and built 7¾ pounds of muscle. His waist measurement shrank from 42½ to 31¾—a reduction of 10¾ inches.

"People at work used to make jokes about my *pregnancy*," cracked Ken in his driest sense of humor. "Finally, I decided it was time to give birth to a new body. Now, these same people are envious, and the joke's on them."

Both Claude and Ken had the patience to continue with the course until they not only reached but also exceeded their goals. It took Claude twelve weeks and Ken fourteen weeks to do so.

Both wanted a flat stomach. But neither, at their ages, was concerned with getting an extremely muscular waist. They did want to maintain their results, however.

The following details should help clarify your goals.

A Few Definitions

Since the title of this book is *A Flat Stomach ASAP,* now is the time to describe what these concepts imply.

Even though *stomach* is technically defined as your primary organ of digestion, it's popularly used to mean the front of your waist. In this book, stomach, belly, middle, and midsection all stand for your frontal waist area.

Flat as a modifier to stomach means straight, primarily as viewed vertically from the side. You have a flat stomach if, when you're seen in a standing pose from the side while wearing a bathing suit, the area between your sternum and a point approximately two inches below your navel forms a straight line. Important: This straight line should be visible with your belly relaxed and not sucked in.

From my research with thousands of overfat people, I've found that with proper Awareness, Science, Application, and Persistence—or simply ASAP—almost anyone can get a flat stomach.

In fact, some of my trainees improve upon that straight line and develop a concave stomach. Achieving a concave stomach requires exceptional genetics, dedication, and attention to detail. The few who succeed are rewarded with abdominal muscles—or abs for short—that are referred to as chiseled, ripped, cut, rock hard, washboards, six-packs, killer, awesome, and perfect.

I like the idea of perfection. But I fully realize that developing perfect abs is an unrealistic goal for most people. And besides, what's perfect anyway? Perfection for me wouldn't be perfection for you.

Instead of perfection, a better goal is to strive toward getting your personal-best look. No one ever built a great body without having personal-best abdominals. And personal-best abdominals begin with a flat stomach.

If you're successful in getting a flat stomach—and with this course I'm confident that you will be—then you may want to try the advanced, personal-best abs routine that is presented in chapter 15.

ASAP Works

It doesn't matter if your goal is simply a flat stomach, or your personal-best abdominals, or something in between—the optimum approach for the look you want is a disciplined dose of Awareness, Science, Application, and Persistence.

ASAP is the way.

Why not get started *as soon as possible?*

2

ANATOMY:

UNDERSTAND YOUR MIDSECTION

For you to conquer your bulging belly you need a basic understanding of what's below the surface of your midsection.

Sure, you already know that your middle contains a backbone, digestive organs, and a few rolls of surface flab. But did you know that your waist also houses numerous hormone-secreting glands, eight major muscles, and billions of energy-storing cells? Being aware of the anatomy and the functions of these tissues will make a big difference in helping you eliminate your protrusion.

And did you know that your skin, that protective covering that stretches from head to belly to toe, is one of the most important factors in achieving a flat stomach? At least it is if you comprehend and apply a long-ignored function of this unique structure.

You're going to learn in this chapter some surprising facts and practical guidelines concerning your skin and other midsection components. So do as one of my favorite teachers used to say—"Put on your thinking cap."

Let's begin your anatomy lesson from the inside out.

Internal Organs

In the upper middle of your waist, tucked under your diaphragm, are your stomach and liver. Slightly under those organs lie your pancreas and spleen. Below your stomach is the small intestine, which twists around in the center of your midsection at navel level and connects to the large intestine or colon. In the same general area are also your kidneys.

Intersecting the bottom of the abdominal region is the pelvic cavity, which houses the internal reproductive organs, the urinary bladder, and the lower parts of the digestive system.

The midsection organs that are related to digestion are the stomach, liver, pancreas, small intestine, and large intestine. The spleen is an important organ in the lymphatic system. The two kidneys are the primary organs of the urinary system along with the bladder. The internal reproductive organs for the female are the ovaries, uterine tubes, and uterus. For the male, the organs on the inside include the prostate and seminal vessels, and on the outside the penis and testes.

Most of these organs contain glands that secrete hormones. Hormones are chemicals that can stimulate, regulate, and inhibit various bodily processes and actions. As you'll see, certain hormones have a role in directing energy consumption, expenditure, and storage.

Influential Hormones

Here's the latest thinking on the hormones that can influence the results of the ASAP program.

Insulin. Insulin is made by the pancreas. Its main function is to drive sugar and fat out of your bloodstream and into cells. The sugar can go into virtually any cell for fuel now or later. Most of the fat goes into your adipose cells for storage.

Insulin is the most powerful profat hormone and the primary promoter of fat preservation. This hormone is a holdover from the Ice Age, when it was an advantage to be able quickly to store as much fat as possible. Ample body fat meant survival when food was scarce. Insulin operates to conserve your fat stores by pushing your body to use sugar for energy instead of fat.

Big meals bring on big insulin responses, which tend to work against someone trying to lose fat. That's why the ASAP eating plan advocates the consumption of small meals. A minimeal, say three hundred calories or less, brings on a small insulin response.

Noradrenaline. This stimulant is produced by your adrenal glands, which are near your kidneys. Noradrenaline causes your body to burn more calories, especially from fat cells.

The adrenal glands secrete noradrenaline under three conditions: cold temperatures, hard exercise, and frequent eating. Practical guidelines, therefore, involve controlling your environment and clothing to reinforce body coolness, performing high-intensity exercise, eating a minimeal every three hours during the day, and sipping ice-cold water almost continuously throughout your waking hours.

Adrenaline. Also manufactured by your adrenal glands, adrenaline mobilizes great surges of energy. It emerges when you're frightened, afraid, or forced to respond quickly. Interestingly, adrenaline automatically speeds up your heart and respiration rates and extinguishes all desire to eat.

Estrogen. Estrogen is the best known female hormone. At and after puberty, appropriate levels of estrogen bring about the deposition of fat in the breasts, hips, and thighs of young women. This powerful chemical influences the physiology of women in many ways throughout their lives. Estrogen is produced not only in the ovaries but also in the fat cells.

Progesterone. This is another female hormone that originates in the ovaries. Both progesterone and estrogen vary in somewhat of an inverse ratio during a normal menstrual cycle. During pregnancy, women have very high levels of progesterone and estrogen, which both accentuate fatness.

Progesterone is catabolic, which means it tends to break down muscle protein. Thus, when it is at its highest levels—usually a day or two before menstruation begins—most women feel sluggish and less motivated to exercise.

Testosterone. The major male hormone, testosterone, is anabolic. This means that it promotes the buildup of muscle protein. Testosterone is produced by the male's testes and, to a much lesser extent, by the adrenal glands of both sexes. Men normally have much higher levels of testosterone than women. High levels of testosterone facilitate fat loss, leanness, and strength building.

Serotonin. This well-publicized chemical is secreted by nerves throughout your body. Research has established a strong relationship between serotonin and hunger. Low levels in the brain initiate hunger, and high brain levels curb hunger and make you feel full. Carbohydrate-rich foods do a good job of elevating serotonin. That's one reason why the ASAP diet provides 60 percent of its calories from carbohydrates.

Cholecystokinin. This interesting hormone is produced by your intestines mainly as fatty foods empty out of the stomach. Once cholecystokinin is secreted, it is picked up by the bloodstream, where it soon makes its way to the hypothalamus, or appetite-control center, in the brain. The end result is a feeling of fullness and satiety.

For any fat-loss diet to be most effective, it must supply a moderate amount of fatty foods daily. Such foods produce cholecystokinin, and cholecystokinin in turn leads to satiety. Fats compose approximately 20 percent of the calories on the ASAP eating plan.

Muscles of the Midsection

Sheathing the internal organs on the front side of your waist are four layered muscles. The back of your waist contains your spine and four more major muscles. All of these muscles support and protect your internal organs, and they help to keep your pelvis and spine in proper alignment.

Let's take a look at each structure.

Transverse abdominis. Of the four front muscles, this one lies innermost to your organs, at least it does until it crosses under your navel. When the lower fibers of this broad, flat, horizontal muscle get below the navel, they form a sheath opening with two other muscles, which permits the rectus abdominis to push through and attach securely to the pubis bone. As the transverse muscles contract, they compress the internal organs. This helps the lungs exhale and the body perform the normal process of elimination.

Internal oblique. This on-the-side muscle lies on top of the transverse abdominis. The muscle fibers start at the hip and run diagonally upward to meet the lower ribs. Lateral flexion and torso rotation to the same side are the main functions of the internal oblique muscles.

External oblique. This wide but thin muscle originates at the borders of the lower ribs and extends forward and downward. The fibers run at right angles to those of the internal oblique. The primary functions of the external oblique are to bend the spine to the same side and to rotate the torso to the opposite side.

Rectus abdominis. This outermost, frontal muscle stretches vertically from the rib cage to the pubis bone. The function of the rectus abdominis is to shorten the distance between the breastbone and the pelvic girdle. A lean individual with well-developed rectus abdominis on each side of the midline can usually display three paired blocks of muscle. These blocks are caused by crossing tendinous inscriptions.

Psoas major, quadratus lumborium, erector spinae, and latissimus dorsi. These four muscles attach to, move, or support your lumbar spine. When the muscles of your lower back are strong, they create a tight protective girdle around the spine. Weak lower back muscles—combined with weak abdominal and oblique muscles—encourage the spine to sag toward the front of the body, which may lead to injury and pain. Strong lower back, abdominal, and oblique muscles help you to maintain a healthy, upright posture—which allows you to look better, feel better, and perform better in sports and recreational activities.

Fat Cells

Intermingled in and around the muscles and organs of your midsection is a yellowish tissue called fat. At body temperature fat is a thick liquid. It feels semisolid in your bulges because the walls of the fat cell keep it in place.

Seen under a microscope, fat cells look like a bubble bath. The globules are grouped together with stringy intercellular glue and streaked with narrow filaments of connective tissue, blood vessels, and nerves. This network of fat cells forms a versatile living inner tube, for the cells can inflate or deflate as required.

EXERCISE CONSIDERATIONS

To organize the most effective exercise routine for the midsection, there are seven considerations that guide me in my research.

- Identify the major muscles that compose the waist.

- Determine the primary function of each muscle.

- Design an exercise to simulate each muscle's primary function.

- Analyze each exercise according to its ability to provide full-range movement.

- Test each exercise with a group of people.

- Evaluate each exercise according to the feedback from those tested.

- Arrange routines of the best exercises and test and evaluate them with groups of people.

After going through this seven-step process with multiple groups of people, I observe definite trends. Gradually, I develop exercise routines that produce the best muscle strenghtening, shaping, and defining.

Throughout your midsection you have billions of fat cells. That's right—billions with a *b*. In fact, scientists have taken samples of fat from throughout the human body and actually counted the number of cells. Although this research is still in its infancy and depends on extrapolation, some interesting findings emerge. Naturally, the number of fat cells can vary greatly from person to person, depending primarily on genetic factors.

Numbers, for example, range from a low of 10 billion to a high of 250 billion. Obviously, a person with a minimum number of fat cells has a lower probability of being fat compared to a person with a high number of fat cells.

Research reveals the average woman in the United States has approximately 42 billion fat cells. The average man has fewer, about 25 billion fat cells.

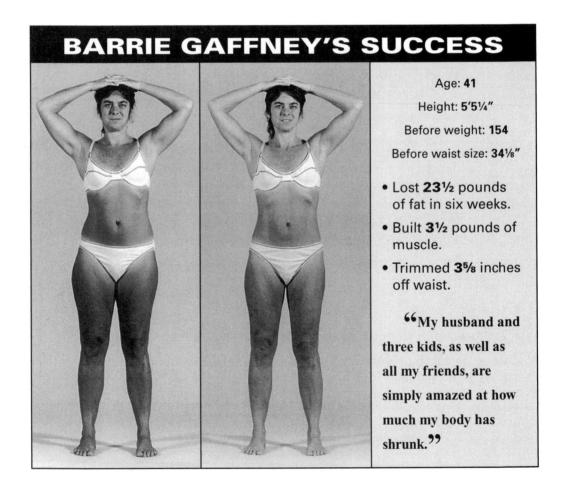

BARRIE GAFFNEY'S SUCCESS

Age: **41**

Height: **5'5¼"**

Before weight: **154**

Before waist size: **34⅛"**

- Lost **23½ pounds** of fat in six weeks.
- Built **3½ pounds of muscle.**
- Trimmed **3⅝ inches** off waist.

"My husband and three kids, as well as all my friends, are simply amazed at how much my body has shrunk."

Interestingly, women tend to deposit fat first on their hips and thighs before it goes on their stomachs. Men, however, put fat on their bellies first. Men usually have greater numbers of fat cells throughout their midsections than do women.

Body fat is composed of 79 percent lipids, 15 percent water, and 6 percent proteins. It is because of the high concentrations of lipids that fat contains so many calories. The 3,500 calories in a pound of fat is almost six times the number of calories in an equal amount of muscle tissue.

Fat is your body's most concentrated way of storing the fuel it needs for energy. Fat also provides insulation, warmth, and protection to your muscles and internal organs. Without such warmth, even a light breeze would send you scurrying for a coat.

Fat is crucial to reproduction as well, which is why women average 68 percent more fat cells than men. Also many female hormones, as discussed earlier, share regulatory relationships with fat cells.

While men, primarily because of their hormones, have somewhat of an advantage in losing fat compared to women, the same physiological facts are applicable to both sexes. Of course, there are certain rules that a woman needs to pay particular attention to, and they will be reinforced at the appropriate time.

Furthermore, even if you are not blessed with the best genetics—which means you may have several times as many fat cells as the average man or woman—you can successfully shrink your fat cells. You can lose significant pounds and inches from your waist and elsewhere.

Yes, you may have a harder time getting lean than does the average man or woman. If that is the case, the ASAP course will teach you how to face the facts head-on by realizing that you'll require extra time and effort to reach your goal. But regardless, you're on solid ground with the ASAP program.

Skin Facts

Few people realize that the skin is their body's largest organ. Surprisingly, an average adult's skin would cover twenty square feet if it were laid out flat. This overall size, or surface area, is the primary reason why as much as 85 percent of the heat you transmit each day emerges through your skin.

Heat loss, in case you didn't know it, is directly related to fat loss.

It's important that you understand the following connection: *Fat throughout your body is energy. Energy is best expressed as calories, which are units of heat measurement.*

One ounce of body fat supplies 219 calories, and one pound contains approximately 3,500 calories.

Your body uses hundreds of calories each day to keep itself functioning. These calories are generated from the foods you consume and from energy-storage spots, such as fat cells. Although your body resorts to several different energy-producing pathways, all of them require calories. Calories count significantly in losing fat.

Heat calories transfer out of your skin by radiation, conduction, convection, and evaporation.

Approximately 50 percent of the calories eliminated through your skin each day are lost as radiant heat. Radiation is why a tall woman has an easier time losing fat than a shorter woman of the same weight. A taller woman has more skin than a shorter woman, and thus she is able to radiate more heat to the environment.

Conduction is the transfer of calories through direct contact. For example, when you get into a cool swimming pool, heat from your body immediately goes into the water. Water is a much better conductor than air, so you can lose more calories in cold water than in cold air. Drinking chilled water is another way to take advantage of conduction, which I'll thoroughly discuss in chapter 6. To be almost shivering, which is another example of conduction, also stimulates your adrenal glands to produce noradrenaline—which in turn causes your body to burn more calories.

Your skin disposes of another 15 percent of heat by convection. This means that air is circulating around your skin to move away the heat. That's why the wind makes you feel cooler when you bicycle or walk. That's why an overhead fan in a workout room can benefit the heat-loss process as you exercise below.

While you may not be aware of it, your skin perspires constantly. This unnoticeable perspiration is eliminated by evaporation. At ordinary room temperatures, the moisture vaporized from your skin, plus that from your lungs, accounts for approximately 25 percent of the calories lost from your body at rest. One-third of heat loss by evaporation is removed through your lungs, and the other two-thirds from invisible perspiration on your skin.

Keeping Your Skin Cool

Few people have ever considered the impact that keeping the skin cool has on the fat-loss process. When I started incorporating this concept into my standard diet and exercise program in 1990, I immediately noticed a significant improvement in average fat loss among these groups compared to previous groups that did not use the technique.

Since then I've continually refined the keeping-cool concept, and I'll cover it in detail in chapters 6 and 8.

Interrelationships

You should now begin to realize the interrelationships among your internal organs, hormones, muscles, fat cells, and skin. Can you see how simply cutting back on your eating and increasing your exercising is not enough, especially if you are serious about *fast* fat loss?

Hormones influence both your muscles and fat cells. And so do eating and exercising. But for maximum fat loss, and because of the interrelationships, the caloric composition of your diet and the way you perform your exercises become salient factors. Plus, let's not forget about the function of your skin and how to facilitate heat loss through keeping cool and drinking plenty of cold water. *A Flat Stomach ASAP* incorporates all of these interrelationships into result-producing guidelines.

The ASAP Approach

It's important to understand that the living inner tube of fatty cells that surround your waist contains too much liquid fat. Your goal is to deflate your inner tube—in the fastest way possible.

To accomplish this goal, you must send the correct signals to your system to give up the calories within your fat cells and transfer them out of your body. The correct signals involve basic applications of anatomy and physiology, which require many complicated interrelationships.

For more than two decades, I've worked at streamlining these interrelationships into specific rules. These rules will be stressed throughout this book.

In general, however, the success of *A Flat Stomach ASAP,* is based on a dynamic formula:

- A simple *eating plan* that gradually reduces calories and emphasizes basic foods. A key guideline is adhering to five minimeals per day.
- A unique *exercising routine* that involves super-slow movement against progressively heavier resistance. Super-slow movement is the fastest way to strengthen, reshape, and define your abdominals and other muscles.

- A powerful *superhydrating schedule* that promotes the continuous sipping of more than one gallon of ice-cold water each day. Superhydration synergizes your eating and exercising to accelerate stomach flattening.

Soon you'll be prepared to incorporate a simple *eating plan,* a unique *exercising routine,* and a powerful *superhydrating schedule* into your daily lifestyle.

Soon your body will be lean and your belly will be flat.

3

ACKNOWLEDGMENT:

EVALUATE YOUR CURRENT CONDITION

You already know if you have a protruding stomach or not. At least you should if you read the definitions at the end of chapter 1. Remember, a flat stomach means that the area from the sternum to below the navel resembles a straight line. If that area rounds or bulges, you are probably overfat.

But how overfat are you? Can you measure it and put a number on your fatness? Yes, and in this chapter I'll describe how to estimate fatness by using a simple test.

What about your body weight? Is it a good way to determine if you're fit and in great shape? Only in a very general way. A better way is to take full-body photographs of yourself and compare them with your weight and your circumference measurements. I'll show you what I mean by this and more in this chapter.

But first, if you haven't already thumbed through this book and examined most of the success stories—which include before-and-after pictures and measurements—I want you to do so now. Keep an eye open for body shapes that are similar to your own. This will help you not only evaluate your current condition but also establish realistic expectations for the ASAP course.

Do not skip the application of this chapter. Take measurements and photographs before you begin the ASAP plan. You'll be glad you did once the pounds and inches start melting away.

The objectives of these procedures are to prompt you to record and recognize your present condition, motivate you to improve, help you to identify your achievements, and increase your knowledge of your body.

The most important quality of your measurements is their accuracy. You must follow the recommended guidelines carefully. Be precise and be consistent.

Measuring Fat

Sure, you can see and feel the rolls of fat around your waist. But how do you put a percentage on the amount of fat you have? Conventional height-weight charts are of little help, since they don't measure fat. Scientific methods that are meaningful include calculations based on X rays, ultrasound waves, underwater weighing, and electrical impedance. These techniques require special equipment and expertise and can be time-consuming and expensive.

I've had good success with using the Lange Skinfold Caliper to measure the thickness of folds of skin and fat in various areas of the body. The method I recommend for taking skin folds and in turn calculating the percentage of body fat comes from work done by William Baum, Michele Baum, and Peter Raven, which was reported in the *Research Quarterly for Exercise and Sport* (52:380–84, 1981). You can probably schedule a skin fold/fat assessment at your local YMCA, fitness center, or university exercise science department.

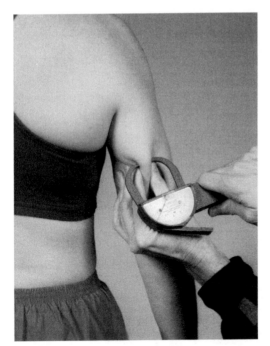

Caliper test: Measurements done with a Lange Skinfold Caliper provide a more accurate method—compared to the pinch test—of determining percentage of body fat.

In the meantime, you can get a fair estimate of your percent body fat by using the pinch test.

Pinch Test

The pinch test for both men and women requires taking two measurements, the first on the back of the upper arm and the second beside the navel. Here's the procedure to follow:

1. Have a friend do the pinching and measuring. It's difficult to pinch your own skin fold accurately.
2. Locate the first skin fold site on the back of the right upper arm (triceps area) midway between the shoulder and elbow. Let the arm hang loosely at the side.
3. Grasp a vertical fold of skin between the thumb and first finger. Pull the skin and fat away from the arm. Make sure the fold includes just skin and fat and no muscle.
4. Measure with a ruler the thickness of the skin to the nearest quarter of an inch. Be sure to measure the distance between the thumb and the finger. Sometimes the outer portion of the fold is thicker than the

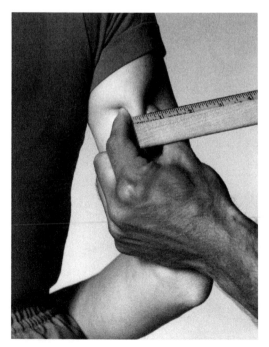

Pinch test: On the back side of the right upper arm, or triceps area, pick up a double layer of skin and measure the vertical thickness with a ruler. A second pinch is taken on the right side of the navel in a vertical position and added to the upper-arm measurement. The total of the two measurements is then converted to an estimated percentage of body fat from the table on page 30.

flesh grasped between the fingers. To avoid this, make sure the fold is level with the side of the thumb. Do not press the ruler against the skin. This will flatten it and make it appear thicker than it really is.

5. Take two separate measurements of the triceps skin fold thickness, releasing the skin between each measure, and record the average of the two.

6. Locate the second skin fold site, which is immediately adjacent to the right side of the navel.

7. Grasp a vertical fold of skin between the thumb and first finger and follow the same technique as previously described.

8. Take two separate measurements of the abdominal skin fold thickness and record the average of the two.

9. Add the average triceps skin fold to the average abdominal skin fold. This is your combined total.

10. Estimate percentage of body fat from the chart below and record it on page 33.

11. Determine total fat loss at the end of the program by multiplying percentage of body fat times body weight for the before-and-after tests. For example, if a woman weighed 140 pounds with 28 percent body fat at the start of the program, that's 39.2 pounds of fat. If she completed the program at 125 pounds and 18 percent body fat, that's 22.5

ESTIMATED PERCENTAGE OF BODY FAT

Skin Fold Thickness Triceps Plus Abdominal	Percent Fat	
	Men	Women
¾ inch	5–9	8–13
1 inch	9–13	13–18
1¼ inches	13–18	18–23
1½ inches	18–22	23–28
1¾ inches	22–27	28–33
2¼ inches	27–32	33–38
2¾ inches	32–37	38–43

pounds of fat. The difference between 39.2 and 22.5 is 16.7 pounds of total fat loss.

12. Calculate the amount of muscle gained by subtracting the weight lost from the total fat lost. In the example above, where fat loss equaled 16.7 pounds and weight loss was 15 pounds, 1.7 pounds of muscle were gained.

Fat composes more than 25 percent of the body weight of most Americans. An ideal amount of body fat for most men is 12 percent. The average healthy woman's ideal status is 18 percent. Lean, athletic men and women may desire to lower their ideal figures by another 5 or 6 percentage points.

Body Weight

It seems rather simple to weigh yourself on a standard bathroom scale. But as many people can attest, strange fluctuations often occur. The problem may have to do with your weighing techniques, your scale, or your body.

Your weighing techniques should be consistent. The scale should rest on a hard flat floor, not on a soft rug or other uneven surface. You should stand in the center of the scale, not in the front or back or to either side. Make sure your weight is equally distributed on both feet and don't hold on to anything during the process.

Time of day is also important, as are the clothes you wear. One appropriate time to weigh is first thing in the morning, after voiding, while completely nude.

A normal bathroom scale usually varies in its weighing by 1 to 2 percent. Some can vary as much as 5 percent. Of course, if you pick it up, move it around, get it wet, jiggle it, drop it, or fiddle excessively with the zeroing dial, then it may be completely unreliable.

The last problem may have to do with dramatic changes that can occur daily, or even hourly, in some individuals' bodies. A few women have been known to gain or lose as many as 5 pounds in a single day, usually as a result of hormones, water retention, and fluid and blood loss. This fluctuation is the primary reason many specialists in the reducing field recommend that you weigh yourself no more than once a week.

Once-a-week weighings are probably too infrequent for most people. Daily weighing is probably too often. I recommend that you weigh yourself three times a week on nonconsecutive days. Weighing yourself on your workout days is a good way to keep a record of your weight.

Circumference Measurements

Circumference measurements are meaningful because they let you know what is happening to specific areas of your body. A flexible sixty-inch tape and a few useful tips are all you need—plus a bathing suit. Both men and women should wear a tight bathing suit that reveals their entire midsection.

I use a plastic measuring tape because, unlike some cloth and paper tapes, it is not subject to shrinking or stretching. It's important to use the same tape for all the measurements.

When taking the measurements, apply the tape lightly to the skin. The tape should be taut but not tight. If you pull the tape too tight, it will compress the soft tissue and make the value smaller than it actually is. Take duplicate measurements to the nearest eighth of an inch at each of the described sites below and use the average figure as the circumference score.

Experience has shown me that people lose fat differently from their waistlines. Some lose fat first from several inches above navel level. Others reduce it first from several inches below navel level. Yet others eliminate it from the navel level first. That's why you need to use three different waist circumferences: two inches above your navel, navel level, and two inches below your navel level. Make the reading at the midpoint of a quiet expiration. Do not pull in the belly. Record the numbers in the chart on page 33.

Note: Throughout this book, in the success stories and for calculation purposes, each person's largest before-and-after difference from the three midsection levels was used as his or her single waist measurement.

Besides the three waist measurements, it is also important to record the circumferences of your hips and upper thighs. Take your hips around the largest protrusion of your buttocks with your heels together. Measure each thigh while in a standing position with the heels a shoulder's width apart and weight equally distributed on both feet. The tape circles just below where the buttocks merge into the back thigh. Again record these numbers in the appropriate place on page 33.

One more thing: It is difficult to take your own measurements accurately. You'll get truer numbers if you have someone else do them for you.

Full-Body Photographs

There is no better way to evaluate the current condition of your midsection than to have full-body photographs taken of yourself in a small, tight bathing suit.

ASAP MEASUREMENTS

Name: _____   Age: _____   Height: _____

Pinch Test	Before	After	Difference
Right triceps	_____	_____	_____
Right abdominal	_____	_____	_____
Combined total	_____	_____	_____
Body fat percent	_____	_____	_____
Fat pounds	_____	_____	_____

Body Weight	Before	After	Difference
	_____	_____	_____
		Total fat lost	_____
		Muscle gained	_____

Circumference	Before	After	Difference
2″ above navel	_____	_____	_____
Waist at navel	_____	_____	_____
2″ below navel	_____	_____	_____
Hips	_____	_____	_____
Right thigh	_____	_____	_____
Left thigh	_____	_____	_____

Most people are not fully aware of their bodies until they see themselves from the front, side, and back in full-body pictures.

Taking full-length photographs like those used in the before-and-after sequences throughout this book is not difficult. But there are some important guidelines that you must apply to make the operation significant. The most important factor is standardization—standardization of the bathing suit, poses, background, film, camera position, and printing.

1. Wear a snug bathing suit (a solid color is best) and stand against an uncluttered, light background. Women should wear a two-piece bathing suit so their waistline is in plain sight.
2. Have your photographer use a 35-millimeter camera and load it with black-and-white print film. Black-and-white film is better than color film because it allows you to concentrate more on your body and less on your clothes and surroundings.
3. Have the photographer move away from you until he can see your entire body in the viewfinder. The camera should be turned sideways for a vertical format negative. He should sit in a chair and hold the camera level with your navel, or better yet, mount the camera at this level on a tripod.

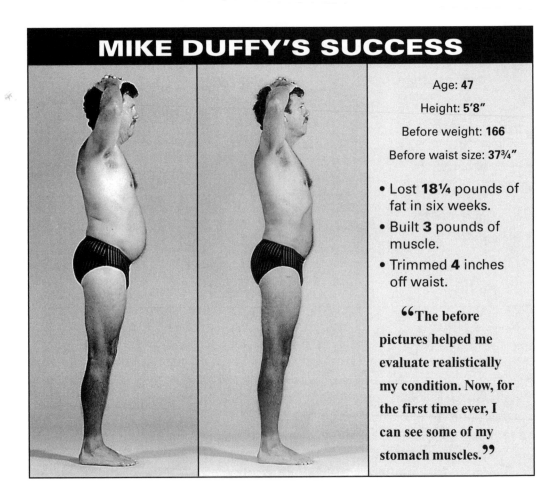

MIKE DUFFY'S SUCCESS

Age: **47**

Height: **5'8"**

Before weight: **166**

Before waist size: **37¾"**

- Lost **18¼** pounds of fat in six weeks.
- Built **3** pounds of muscle.
- Trimmed **4** inches off waist.

"The before pictures helped me evaluate realistically my condition. Now, for the first time ever, I can see some of my stomach muscles."

4. Stand relaxed and have three pictures taken from three different positions—front, right side, and back. Place your hands on top of your head for all three pictures. Your heels should be eight inches apart for the front and back poses, but place them together in the side shot. Do not try to suck in your belly in any of the pictures. Stay relaxed.

5. Process the film and get two prints made of each negative. On the backs of each photograph in both sets write the date and your weight. File one set for safekeeping.

6. Select the least attractive photograph of the remaining set. Carry it around in your billfold or pocketbook or put it on your refrigerator door. Look at it often. Be determined to reduce and improve.

7. Repeat the picture-taking session in six weeks, or after you complete the ASAP course. Wear the same bathing suit and assume the same poses and procedures. *Note:* You may need to use clothespins on your old bathing suit to make it fit snugly.

8. Instruct the photo processor to make your after prints exactly the same size as your before prints. *Important:* Your height in all the before-and-after photos must be standarized for valid comparisons to be made and fat and inch losses to be noted. This is done by comparison cropping at the processing lab.

Realistic Goals

Taking your body-fat and circumference measurements will help you determine realistic goals for your ASAP program. The success stories throughout this book will also help.

The following averages provide specific pounds and inches lost. They were compiled from the before-and-after measurements of 150 people (41 men and 109 women) who have been through one or more of the phases of the *A Flat Stomach ASAP* course. Most of these people completed the program in 1996 under my supervision at the Gainesville Health & Fitness Center in Gainesville, Florida.

Each man lost an average of:
- 23 pounds of fat
- 4 inches off the waist
- 2¼ inches off the hips
- 3½ inches off the thighs

Each woman lost an average of:
- 15 pounds of fat
- 3½ inches off the waist
- 2¼ inches off the hips
- 4 inches off the thighs

The same men added an average of 4 pounds of muscle to their physiques. The women gained slightly less muscle at 3½ pounds average per woman.

These numbers provide realistic goals for most men and women motivated to follow the six-week ASAP course. Some individuals will achieve lower results and some can achieve greater results—as much as 50 percent above some of the averages.

The Bottom Line

Estimating skin fold readings, percent body fat, total fat lost, muscle gained, and circumference measurements, and taking full-body photos can be somewhat complicated and perplexing. But in the final analysis, here's the bottom line:

- If your belly bulges when you are standing, or hangs over your belt when you're sitting, *or*
- If you simply want to lose pounds and inches from your waistline, *or*
- If you want abdominal muscle sharpness instead of smoothness, *then*

You are a prime participant for *A Flat Stomach ASAP*.

SCIENCE

Part Two

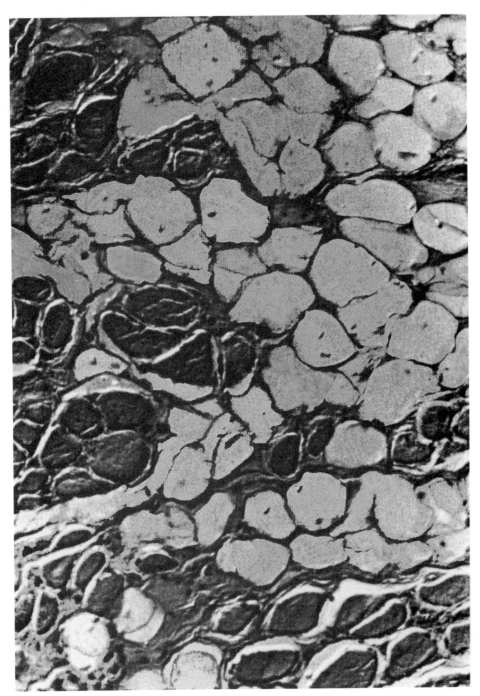

The two most changeable components of the body are fat and muscle. This photograph shows a microscopic cross section of fat cells (light colored) and muscle cells (dark colored), which are intermingled throughout the midsection. With the proper application of the rules governing satiation, strength, superhydration, sleep, and synergy, fat cells shrink and muscle cells expand. This compounded effect produces a harder, smaller, and flatter stomach.

4

SATIATION:

EAT YOUR FAT AWAY

Satiation means to satisfy completely. In relation to food it implies eating to the point that all desire is lost. Satiation in many peoples' minds requires leaving the dinner table feeling thoroughly stuffed.

I understand that stuffed feeling. For most of my teenage years I was a skinny athlete. But I desperately wanted to be bigger so I could play sports better. Eating large amounts of food each day, or so I thought, was a good way to get bigger. I was particularly attracted to those "all you can eat" cafeterias and restaurants. At such establishments, I would stuff myself with a large array of foods and always try to force one more piece of pie into my mouth.

I remember well that sensation of overfullness throughout my body as I walked from the cafeteria to the car. All I wanted to do was get home and take a long nap.

Most of you have experienced that same stuffed feeling. You may have felt it not only during your teenage years but even now, at special celebrations and holidays—such as Thanksgiving and Christmas.

But why do we continue to glut our bellies with excessive foods, especially since we are bombarded with national guidelines to eat less fat and sugar and fewer calories? Understanding the answer to this question is one of the keys to applying the proper diet to shrink your fat cells.

Satiation and Survival

Through most of the history of humankind, living was hard. As humans migrated out of Africa more than 100,000 years ago, things got even harder. Snow and ice were often part of the climate, and humans had to adapt or die.

One way that prehistoric men and women adapted was by getting fatter. Scientists know that animals in cold climates tend to be fatter than those in warm environments. This is as true for humans as it is for polar bears and whales.

Our Ice Age ancestors survived by learning to store fat. It helped them keep warm, it gave them a portable food supply when vegetation was absent and game was scarce, and it helped women survive pregnancy and childbirth. Thin people were inclined to die out, while those who were fatter tended to reproduce and survive.

But how did our ancestors actually learn to store fat? Perhaps simply by observing that those who thoroughly gorged themselves in times of feast tended to get fatter than those who did not. A stuffed stomach produced satiation, satiation improved fat storage, and fat storage increased the probability of survival.

Thus over hundreds of generations a preference for fatness was bred into the genes of humankind.

Even though times have changed greatly, the heredity bias for fatness is still very much alive and well in today's society. It was only twelve thousand years ago that the last Ice Age finally waned in northern Europe, a mere second or two on the evolutionary time clock.

Rather than allow our genes' bias for fatness to assume more control over our lives, a better alternative is to understand it and, in turn, use this information to help us attack and conquer the situation. That's precisely what I've been doing for many years.

It should now be fairly obvious that our attraction to feasting excessively is primarily genetic. But it should also be equally obvious—especially from a review of chapter 2—that science can provide a lot of ammunition concerning satiation, fat storage, and fat loss.

Three salient issues are the length, composition, and frequency of meals.

Length of Meals

After a moderate amount of food enters your stomach, it takes twenty minutes for appropriate hormones to circulate and reach your brain's appetite-control mechanism. Loss of desire to eat, or satiation, is the result.

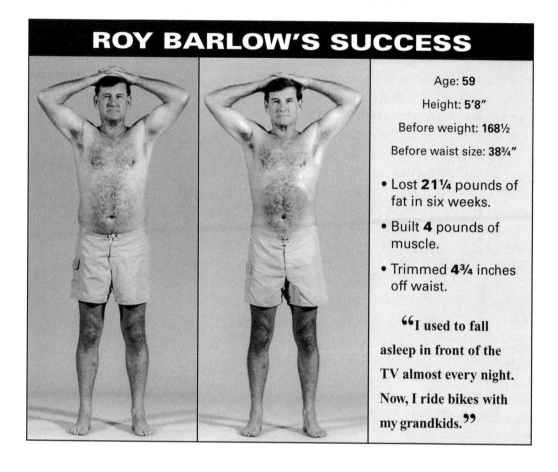

ROY BARLOW'S SUCCESS

Age: **59**

Height: **5'8"**

Before weight: **168½**

Before waist size: **38¾"**

- Lost **21¼** pounds of fat in six weeks.
- Built **4** pounds of muscle.
- Trimmed **4¾** inches off waist.

"I used to fall asleep in front of the TV almost every night. Now, I ride bikes with my grandkids."

If you are trying to store fat by consuming excessive calories, it would be to your advantage to eat your food quickly. Wolf down your densest calorie-rich foods in the first ten minutes. That would leave you another ten minutes to focus on accessories and desserts before satiation sets in.

On the other hand, if your goal is to lose fat, then you want to linger over or stretch your meals—especially if your meals are relatively moderate in size. Take small bites. Put your fork down often. Chew your food thoroughly. Drink water frequently.

Most of all, understand that you're probably going to feel hungry until the appetite-control center in your brain gets the correct message. That requires twenty minutes.

Composition of Meals

Calorie-containing foods are classified as carbohydrates, proteins, and fats. An average mixed meal of approximately a thousand calories would be processed in the stomach in two to four hours. A pint of mushy liquid may start exiting the stomach into the small intestines in just ten or fifteen minutes, and a certain amount of water and sugar may be absorbed right through the stomach's walls, but most of what you eat remains in the stomach for several hours.

Carbohydrates eaten alone will exit the stomach faster than proteins. Proteins eaten alone will move on faster than fats, which trigger a hormone that slows the stomach's action. A mixture of carbohydrates, proteins, and fats will remain in the stomach longer than any of these alone. But it is abnormal for any meal to hang in the stomach for more than seven hours. Roughage or fiber is an exception.

Plant fibers—which are technically classified as carbohydrates—consist of leaves, stems, and seeds. They supply indigestible bulk to the diet and help make the system function properly. Because of their indigestibility, some fibers—such as spinach and lettuce—may remain in the stomach for twenty-four hours.

Thus, fibers in your diet slow the movement of food through your stomach and make you feel fuller longer. Once they exit the stomach, they help keep the contents of the intestines moist and easy to eliminate.

It should be evident that humans function best when they have carbohydrates, fats, and proteins—all in adequate amounts. But what is adequate? And what is optimum?

A recent dietary survey revealed that the typical adult in the United States had the following breakdown of calories: 46 percent from carbohydrates, 37 percent from fats, and 17 percent from proteins.

Most nutrition scientists would agree that the typical American's diet could be improved by consuming more carbohydrates and fewer fats.

After working over the last twenty-five years with thousands of men and women who wanted to reduce fat, I've found that what works best is a 60:20:20 breakdown each day. That's 60 percent of calories from carbohydrates, 20 percent from fats, and 20 percent from proteins. This is a composition that is ideal for fat reduction, and it also works well for overall health and fitness.

I've talked with many women who believe that meticulously counting their grams of fat and having it total under ten grams per day is a must for fat-loss success. This is false. Moderate levels of fat per day produce more effective fat loss than very low levels. The primary reason goes back to the fact that fatty

FOOD GROUPS

For many years I taught the four basic food groups to all my dieters. It was a good method for stressing balance and variety in eating. It did, however, place too much emphasis on meat and dairy products.

In 1991, the U.S. Department of Agriculture introduced an improved plan that centers around a Food Guide Pyramid. Instead of four food groups, there are now six. Fruits and vegetables are now separate groups, and a new group called fats, oils, and sweets has been added. The enclosed Simplified Food Guide attaches more importance to breads, vegetables, and fruits than to meat and dairy.

The ASAP eating plan is based on this system. You'll be getting most of your calories from carbohydrates, with only moderate to low amounts of proteins and fats.

Simplified Food Guide

Fats, Oils, and Sweets: use sparingly
Milk, Yogurt, and Cheese Group: 2–3 servings
Meat, Poultry, Fish, Dry Beans, Eggs, and Nut Group: 2–3 servings
Fruit Group: 2–4 servings
Vegetable Group: 3–5 servings
Bread, Cereal, Rice, and Pasta Group: 6–11 servings

Serving Sizes:

Breads and Cereals: A single serving = 1 slice of bread, 1 ounce of ready-to-eat cereal, 4 to 6 small crackers, or ½ cup cooked cereal, rice, or pasta.
Vegetables: A single serving = 1 cup raw leafy vegetables, ½ cup other vegetables (cooked or chopped raw), or ¾ cup vegetable juice.
Fruit: A single serving = 1 medium apple, banana, or orange; ½ cup chopped, cooked, or canned fruit; or ¾ cup juice.
Meat, Poultry, Fish, Dry Beans, Eggs, and Nuts: A single serving = 2 to 3 ounces cooked lean meat, poultry, or fish. For example, ½ chicken breast, 1 chicken leg plus 1 thigh, 1 pork chop, 1 small meat patty, or any lean meat the size of a deck of cards. A half-cup of cooked dry beans, 1 egg, and 1 tablespoon of peanut butter each count as 1 ounce lean meat.
Milk, Yogurt, Cheese: A single serving = 1 cup milk or yogurt, 1½ ounces natural cheese, or 2 ounces processed cheese.

foods stimulate cholecystokinin, the hormone that helps produce satiation. In the ASAP diet, approximately twenty-five grams of fat are in each daily meal schedule for women.

Furthermore, it's important to remember that serotonin—another satiation-producing hormone—is influenced by carbohydrates. That's another reason why each meal on the ASAP eating plan is carbohydrate rich.

Frequency of Meals

If your goal was to get as fat as possible, it would be to your advantage to eat one very large meal each day and then go to sleep.

Who in their right mind, however, would want to practice such a routine?

In reality, many middle-aged businessmen have eating habits that are quite similar to this example. It's a pattern of—no time for breakfast, work through the lunch hour, eat a big dinner, and snack nonstop until bedtime.

Millions of men deprive their bodies when they most need calories and stuff themselves when they'll be doing nothing more strenuous than reading the newspaper and watching television. Such dietary habits make no sense, unless you're trying to expand your fat cells.

Research shows that shrinking fat cells in the most efficient manner requires just the opposite—eating smaller meals more often. Large meals of several thousand calories stimulate excessive insulin production, and you should recall that insulin is your body's most powerful fat-storing hormone. Small meals bring on small insulin responses. Thus, it's advantageous to eat a series of smaller-than-average meals, or more precisely—minimeals.

A minimeal does not have to include a serving from each of the standard food groups. It can be made up of only one or two. It can include all of these food groups in very small amounts. Even a snack can be called a minimeal. Each minimeal should contain from fifty to five hundred calories.

The idea is to spread your calories into five minimeals a day for efficient fat loss. The goal is to have no longer than three to four hours between the eating episodes.

Besides the length, composition, and frequency of meals, there is one more factor that is important to satiation and fat loss. That factor is the total number of calories that you consume each day.

Calorie Allowance

You probably already know that one gram of carbohydrate and one gram of protein each contain four calories, while one gram of fat supplies nine calories. Fat is indeed a potent and necessary source of energy.

To lose body fat effectively and efficiently, you must significantly reduce your daily dietary calories. And to do so, you must monitor your calories—at least for the first several weeks, or until you become accustomed to the appropriate measurements and serving sizes.

Your reduction in calories, however, should not be too low, or your body may pull nutrients from your muscles, and that's not desirable. The majority of the people I've worked with achieve optimum results by adhering to daily calorie levels which range from 1,000 to 1,500. Women respond best to 1,000 to 1,300 calories a day. Men require slightly more, approximately 1,200 to 1,500 calories per day. A slight variation in the total number of daily calories on a weekly basis is also helpful.

Satiation and Science

Satiation doesn't have to mean feeling thoroughly stuffed when you leave the meal table. It can mean being comfortably satisfied, even if you'd rather have more servings of certain foods.

By consuming the appropriate number of daily calories—combined with knowledge of the length, composition, and frequency of meals—you'll be well armed with science to eat your fat away.

5

STRENGTH:

FIRM YOUR FLABBY MUSCLES

Muscles can be strong, shapely, and firm. Or muscles can be weak, stringy, and flabby.

The muscles of most adults in the United States, unfortunately, tend to fall into the latter category. As a result of this degression of the system's underlying support, most people display jiggling flesh throughout their bellies, buttocks, and thighs. But this physical condition doesn't have to stay this way. Corrective action can remedy the situation—and quickly.

Muscles operate under the *use it or lose it* rule. If you work harder this week than you did last week, your involved muscles grow slightly stronger. If you don't work as hard this week as you did last week, then a small amount of shrinkage or wasting away occurs.

Research on Muscle

Studies by Dr. Gilbert Forbes of the University of Rochester School of Medicine reveal that the average man and woman lose one-half pound of muscle per year between the ages of twenty and fifty. Such a process is called *disuse atrophy.*

Losing one-half pound of muscle per year doesn't sound like much, but continued for thirty years, it becomes fifteen pounds. Fifteen pounds of muscle takes up about as much space as two gallon jugs of water, so the overall effect is significant.

"Hold on a second," you may be thinking, "I thought most adults get heavier, not lighter, as they get older?"

You're right. Their overall weight gets heavier, but their muscle mass gets lighter. Which means that something else inside their bodies must not only make up the difference but exceed the weight of the shrinking muscles. That something else, of course, is fat.

While most adults are losing one-half pound of muscle each year, at the same time they are gaining 1½ pounds of fat. Over thirty years, that's a fifteen-pound muscle loss combined with a forty-five-pound fat gain, which amounts to a thirty-pound increase in body weight.

Research on Metabolism

Losing muscle and gaining fat have major influences on metabolism. Your resting metabolism is the number of calories your body requires to function in a relaxed, resting state. Your brain and internal organs—such as your heart, lungs, liver, and kidneys—require a lot of energy. But it's your skeletal muscles, which comprise from 30 to 50 percent of an average person's body weight, that use the most energy.

Add a pound of muscle to your body, and your resting metabolic rate goes up approximately 37.5 calories per day. Lose a pound of muscle through disuse atrophy and the opposite happens: Your rate is lowered by 37.5 calories per day.

Interestingly, a pound of fat also has a metabolic rate: approximately 2 calories per day. Muscle is 18.75 times as active metabolically as the same amount of fat.

You may have noticed that it is more difficult to shed excess fat now than it was when you were younger. Long-term metabolic studies reveal that an average individual experiences a 0.5 percent reduction in resting metabolic rate each year between twenty and fifty years of age. The gradual loss of muscle mass each year is primarily responsible for the metabolic slowdown.

Furthermore, the continued loss of muscle is likely to manifest itself in physical ailments such as lower-back pain, bothersome knees and shoulders, arthritis, or even heart disease. From there, it's often a steady downward spiral.

Atrophy, the shrinkage of tissue, involves the metabolic breakdown of muscle into its constituent compounds, which are removed by the bloodstream. Muscle fibers that atrophy simply lose their fluids and become smaller, weaker, and less supportive.

But your body doesn't have to degenerate this way. You can put a stop to the regression and actually reverse the process. You can rebuild your atrophied muscle with proper strength training.

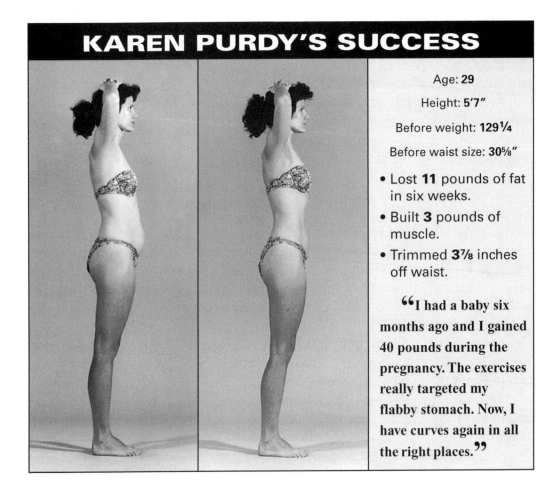

KAREN PURDY'S SUCCESS

Age: **29**

Height: **5'7"**

Before weight: **129¼**

Before waist size: **30⅝"**

- Lost **11** pounds of fat in six weeks.
- Built **3** pounds of muscle.
- Trimmed **3⅞** inches off waist.

"I had a baby six months ago and I gained 40 pounds during the pregnancy. The exercises really targeted my flabby stomach. Now, I have curves again in all the right places."

What Is Proper Strength Training?

Unlike *exercise,* which is a general term applied to almost any type of movement activity, from archery and bowling to walking and yachting, *strength training* requires a specific definition.

I define strength training as movement against resistance to develop the body's muscular structures. From this definition you can evaluate any strength-training endeavor by examining two factors: the quantity of the movement by a specific part of the body and the quality of the resistance applied against it. In fact, I've utilized these two factors in designing the ASAP strength-training routine that I'll describe and illustrate in later chapters.

For the first half of the twentieth century, strength training was known as weight lifting. Later it was modified to weight training and progressive resistance exercise. With the media's help, it has more recently been called "pumping iron."

Generally, all of these names refer to the same thing: movement against resistance. Throughout this book, however, I'll stay with strength training.

Resistance, as the definition stresses, is an important aspect of strength training. Your muscles will not become stronger, firmer, and more shapely unless they are subjected to resistance, or an overload. Once they are overloaded correctly, a chemical reaction takes place within the body that causes the muscles to become stronger.

According to the laws of physics every movement you perform is counteracted by some kind of resistance—even though much of that resistance may be poor in quality. For example, walking is met by air, swimming is slowed by water, and jumping is deterred by gravity. Moving your body weight against air, water, or gravity is not an efficient way to overload your system.

Adding resistance to your arms, legs, torso, and other body parts offers a much more efficient way to overload the muscles. Usually this is accomplished with weights or metal discs that are loaded on bars. The long bars are called barbells and the short ones are dumbbells. Over the last several decades, strength training has become more complex with the additional use of many types of sophisticated machines. For busy people at home, however, neither barbells nor machines are necessary. Strength training can be simplified by using common household items to furnish resistance. Plastic bottles, cans, and other items can work surprisingly well—especially if you master the ASAP style of strength training.

The ASAP style of strength training, which has worked so well for people in this book, is called *super slow.*

Super Slow Described

If you want superfast results from strength training, you must understand and apply super slow.

Super slow means taking fifteen seconds to perform a single repetition. That's right, fifteen seconds! To comprehend how deliberate that is, many trainees typically do ten repetitions in fifteen seconds.

Mastering the super-slow style of strength training is one of the secrets behind the success of *A Flat Stomach ASAP.* Since the super-slow concept is probably new to you, I want to back up a little and fill you in on how it evolved.

The primary person behind super-slow strength training is Ken Hutchins. Ken and I are longtime friends. We trained together in the 1960s in my garage gym in Conroe, Texas. Later in the 1970s and 1980s, Ken and I worked at Nautilus Sports/Medical Industries in Florida. During that time, we planned and conducted—along with Ken's wife, Brenda—many successful diet and exercise programs.

In 1980 we were visited by Vince Bocchicchio, the owner of a large fitness center in New York. Vince had been experimenting with a very slow lifting and lowering protocol with his Nautilus machines. He suggested that we try a ten-second lifting and a ten-second lowering on each repetition. Vince said he had been successfully using this form with many of his members.

Ken and I had both previously employed a very slow form of Nautilus training, which was called negative only. In negative only, a heavier weight than you could normally lift was loaded onto a Nautilus machine. A couple of spotters would lift the weight (or do the positive phase) for you. Then they would transfer the load to your body, which would allow you to do only the lowering (or negative phase). The lowering was performed very slowly in ten seconds.

Negative-only training proved to be an effective mode of strength building. But there were some drawbacks. First, you had to have access to a couple of spotters to lift the weight for you. Second, because people are much stronger negatively than positively, it was moderately possible to injure yourself by using too much resistance on a machine.

We considered Bocchicchio's idea and even tried it on a few machines, but both of us felt that the negative phase was too easy. Eventually, we dismissed Vince's very slow lifting and lowering protocol.

Ken and I believed at that time that the best way to perform a repetition was two seconds in the positive or lifting phase, and four seconds in the negative or lowering phase. That was two seconds up and four seconds down, or approximately six seconds on each repetition. This style became well known as the standard Nautilus protocol.

Several years later, a unique research project forced Ken to reexamine the standard Nautilus protocol. Nautilus Sports/Medical Industries funded a large-scale osteoporosis study in Gainesville, Florida, and Ken and Brenda were responsible for strength training hundreds of women. Early on Ken recognized that many of these older women, especially those in their sixties and seventies, exhibited poor motor control in their lower bodies when applying the standard protocol. Two seconds up and four seconds down per repetition was simply too fast for their neuromuscular systems to perform safely.

Out of necessity, Ken slowed their movements, especially the positive lifting phase, where most of the jerking, twisting, and dangerous actions occurred.

Eventually, he settled on a protocol of ten seconds positive and five seconds negative—or fifteen seconds per repetition.

Ken named this new training style Super Slow®, and eventually he registered his trademark. The super-slow protocol quickly solved the control and safety problems the women involved in the osteoporosis project were having. Furthermore, it allowed Ken and Brenda to better load the muscles, which meant improved strength-training results.

After learning about Ken's progress with super-slow training, I put several male bodybuilders and football players through the 10:5 protocol for six weeks. It's difficult to get experienced trainees to reduce the weight lifted on each machine, which they must do initially to move slowly. Once they all made the transition, however, their results were even better than I had anticipated.

Since then, I have personally supervised thousands of people through various training programs that applied super-slow techniques. Very simply, it's the best way to strength train.

Why Super Slow Works

I visited my first strength-training gym in 1959. Now almost forty years later, I've toured hundreds of gyms and fitness centers throughout the United States. And I have been in gyms in Canada, Mexico, Germany, Great Britain, Australia, Hong Kong, and a few other countries.

But I don't think I've ever been in a gym—with one or two possible exceptions—where the following was *not* happening: *at least 99 percent of the people who were working out were performing their repetitions too fast for best results.* Simply getting these people to do each repetition half as fast as they normally do would automatically improve their results. Reducing the speed by another 50 percent would make the results even more significant.

Why is it so difficult, however, to get most people to slow down their repetitions?

The simple answer is that slowing down the repetition makes the movement harder, and most people want easier, not harder, exercise. Most people feel that they can make progress by getting stronger, which they assume they can achieve by introducing excessive momentum into their lifting and lowering. This excessive momentum then allows them to do more repetitions with greater weight. Yes, they may be able to do more repetitions with greater weight using such a style, but their true strength will test the same or even less.

Super slow prevents this lack of progress. Super-slow training is effective because it eliminates excessive momentum, which occurs when you perform fast, jerky repetitions.

If you begin a repetition with a sudden jerk, then the moving weight can actually pull your body along until you have to catch the weight, which is now in the top position. Such fast, jerky lifting contributes to disproportionate, unbalanced strength development. It neglects many muscle fibers and overstresses others. It is dangerous and can cause injury.

Slow, smooth, concentrated repetitions, on the other hand, recruit a maximum number of muscle fibers, which is a key to effectiveness. And, once again, super-slow repetitions are much safer than faster styles of strength training.

Doing a Super-Slow Repetition

Since this book centers around the midsection, let me describe how to do several repetitions on one of the recommended exercises: the trunk curl. Read the directions first, then sit down on the floor and give this movement a try.

- Lie faceup on the floor.
- Spread your knees and bring the soles of your feet together near your buttocks.
- Place your arms, with your elbows extended, in front of your stomach and interlace your fingers.

This is your starting position with your knees bent and spread, your hands in front of your midsection, and your head and shoulders resting on the floor. Now, do the following very deliberately:

- Think about lifting your head and shoulders off the floor by smoothly tightening your abdominal muscles. Don't actually move your head and shoulders, just think about doing it.
- Concentrate now on lifting your head and shoulders only a barely perceptible one-eighth inch.
- Proceed slowly and smoothly a quarter inch, then half an inch, then one inch.
- Reach with your hands through your thighs, at the same time as you are lifting your shoulders. Your goal is to shorten, as much as possible, the distance between your sternum and navel.
- Continue to curl your shoulders and head up and forward. With your knees bent, your range of motion will be limited to only one-third of a standard sit-up.

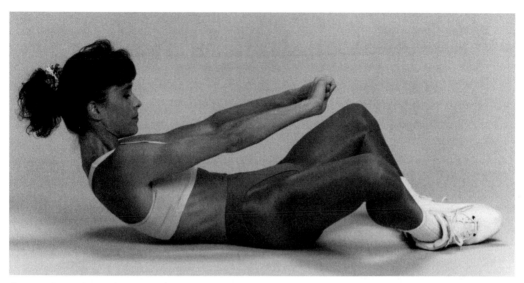

Super-slow trunk curl, top position: Gently roll your head, neck, and shoulders off the floor until your abdominals are tightly contracted.

- Keep your feet stable, eyes open, and face relaxed and breathe normally. Do not hold your breath.
- Try to reach the highest position with your shoulders completely off the floor at about the ten-second mark. Someone with a watch that has a second hand should help you with the counting.
- Pause briefly in the top position.
- Ease out of the top position gradually, and lower your shoulders smoothly to the starting position in five seconds.
- Feel your shoulders and head come in contact with the floor, but do not relax or rest. You want to touch, then barely move again in the upward direction.
- Focus on keeping your head, shoulders, and hands moving at a near-constant speed. Do not try to jerk or heave your head or shoulders suddenly.
- Keep the lifting slow but steady—and the lowering smooth.
- Stop after you've performed three repetitions.

After only three super-slow trunk curls, you should feel a burning sensation in your midsection muscles. Don't be alarmed. The burning sensation is an indication that the involved muscles are being thoroughly worked—for perhaps the first time ever.

Super-Slow Rules

Super slow is definitely the best way to train your abdominal muscles. But there's no reason why you can't use it throughout your body. Super slow can be applied to almost any type of strength-training equipment: home exercise equipment including abdominal rollers, fitness club machines, barbells, dumb-bells, and even your own body weight. Carefully study the following basic guidelines:

1. Perform three to five exercises for your lower body and five to seven exercises for your upper body, and no more than nine exercises in any workout.
2. Train no more than three nonconsecutive days per week. Super-slow strength training necessitates a recovery period of at least forty-eight hours. Your body gets stronger during rest, not during exercise.
3. Select a resistance for each exercise that allows the performance of be-tween four and eight slow repetitions.
   - Begin with a weight at which you can comfortably do four repetitions.
   - Stay with that weight until eight or more strict repetitions are per-formed. In your next workout, increase the resistance by 5 percent.
   - Attempt to increase the number of repetitions, the amount of weight, or both. But do not sacrifice form in an attempt to produce repetition and resistance improvements.
4. Concentrate on each repetition by lifting the weight slowly in ten sec-onds, and by lowering it smoothly in five seconds.
5. Move more slowly, never faster, if in doubt about the speed of move-ment.
6. Relax body parts that are not involved in each exercise. Pay special at-tention to relaxing your face, neck, and hand muscles.
7. Breathe normally. Try not to hold your breath during any repetition.
8. Keep accurate records—date, resistance, repetitions, and overall training time—of each workout.

Great Results As Soon As Possible

Can you now imagine what it would feel like to work not only your midsection but also your lower body and your upper body in the super-slow manner? Talk about getting a superb workout—there's none better.

But because super-slow movements are so thorough, all you need to do is one set of four to eight repetitions. And because an exercise is so intense, you must progress into your routine gradually. That's why initially on the ASAP program, you'll do only five exercises. Eventually, you'll work up to nine exercises. No workout should ever last longer than thirty minutes.

I can promise you, however, that this deliberate, hard, brief style of strength training will force your muscles to become stronger, firmer, and more defined—faster—than you ever thought was possible.

6

SUPERHYDRATION:

EXPERIENCE SOMETHING NEW

1. Ignore
2. Ridicule
3. Attack
4. Copy
5. Steal

According to Arthur Jones, the inventor of Nautilus exercise equipment, the listing above is the pattern of behavior from the so-called experts when a new idea is presented to them.

First, they will ignore the idea because they did not discover it. Second, if the idea persists, they will ridicule it. Third, if the idea stands up to their ridicule, they will attack it. Fourth, if the idea survives their attacks, they will try to copy it. Fifth, faced with the obvious success that has thrived in spite of their efforts, they will remember that the original idea was really theirs in the first place. In other words, the so-called experts eventually will steal the idea and claim it as their own.

Repeatedly throughout his adult life, Jones has seen the experts use this pattern of behavior when considering his work. I observed this firsthand as director of research for Nautilus Sports/Medical Industries for more than seventeen years.

In the early 1970s, Nautilus equipment was ignored, ridiculed, and attacked. Jones, however, was successful at combating these behaviors, and Nautilus equipment gained popularity throughout the world—primarily because it worked; it actually did what it claimed to do.

By 1980, several companies were copying almost everything Nautilus was manufacturing. By 1987, when Jones sold Nautilus, more than twenty-five companies were copying Nautilus machines and violating Jones's patents. Furthermore, at least five exercise experts had already stepped forward and "remembered" that they had invented Jones's machines, or at least the idea they were based on, before he did.

Presenting Superhydration

Superhydration, the concept of sipping one gallon or more of ice-cold water each day, is new, and most importantly—it works.

While I didn't invent the drinking of large amounts of cold water, I was probably the first person to popularize it by connecting it to my fat-loss courses. And I was the first author to provide specific directions on why, how, and when to consume the fluid.

My superhydration idea began to formalize in 1985 as I supervised three large groups of people through the Nautilus diet program in Gainesville, Florida. I continued refining the techniques in Dallas, Texas, when I worked on other fat-loss studies—which were published as *The Six-Week Fat-to-Muscle Makeover, 32 Days to a 32-Inch Waist,* and *Two Weeks to a Tighter Tummy.* Finally, I returned to the Gainesville Health & Fitness Center in Florida, where over the last six years I've had good success with such programs as *Living Longer Stronger, Body Defining,* and *A Flat Stomach ASAP.*

There is no doubt in my mind that superhydration facilitates fat loss in a number of ways, as you'll see in the remainder of this chapter. But there are experts who have *ignored, ridiculed,* and *attacked* my superhydration recommendations.

Superhydration Attacks

In January of 1995, a major story was written on superhydration and my *Living Longer Stronger* book by a reporter for the *Charlotte Observer.* The story was "killed" the night before publication when their expert health advisor determined that "people can't drink one gallon of cold water a day without getting sick . . . and his clinical studies are weak."

A similar situation occurred a month later when the *Los Angeles Times* interviewed me about my superhydration guidelines. On the advice of their experts, they, too, after much consideration, backed off.

It's true that my studies are not performed with large groups in medical clinics or hospitals. They are conducted in commercial fitness centers with small groups of people. But that doesn't make what I do weak. In fact, dealing with small numbers gives me an advantage because I can better supervise the participants and better control many of the variables. And working with individuals in a fitness club, as opposed to a medical environment, is more of a real-life occurrence.

If these newspaper health advisors had bothered examining my published books over the last ten years, they would have seen that *549* women and *271* men have been through at least one of my programs that involved superhydration. Moreover, not a single participant has ever suffered from any major medical problem or side effect as a result of drinking at least one gallon of ice-cold water each day for the duration of the course.

But regardless of what certain experts and advisors have to say about my superhydration ideas, let's back up for a while and look at some of the elementary reasons that you need water.

Water and the Human Body

The human body is from 50 to 65 percent water. But not all body parts have the same water percentage. For example, your blood is 90 percent water, your bone is 30 percent, your brain is 75 percent, your muscle is 72 percent, your fat is 15 percent, and your skin is 71 percent.

Men generally have more water in their bodies than women, primarily because men have more muscle mass and less fat than women. A lean man with a body weight of 180 pounds may have more than 14 gallons of water in his system. A gallon of water weighs slightly more than 8 pounds, so simple multiplication (8×14) reveals that at least 112 pounds of this man's body is water.

You may not think of water as food, but it's the most critical nutrient in your daily life. You can live only a few days without it. Every process in your body requires water. For example, it:

- Makes food digestion possible.
- Acts as a solvent for minerals, vitamins, amino acids, and glucose.
- Carries nutrients through the system.
- Lubricates the joints.
- Serves as a shock absorber inside the eyes and spinal cord.
- Maintains body temperature.

- Rids the body of waste products through the urine.
- Eliminates heat through the skin, lungs, and urine.
- Keeps the skin supple.
- Assists muscular contraction.

Water contributes to so many functions that most people take it for granted. At the end of a long workday, maybe you have a headache. Plus, your eyes are irritated, your back hurts, and your entire body has a dull numbness. You blame it on stress and lack of sleep over the last several nights.

Maybe you're right. But more likely, you're simply suffering from dehydration.

Perhaps you had several cups of coffee for breakfast, a high-fat lunch with more coffee or maybe an alcoholic drink or two, and spent the rest of your time breathing air-conditioned or heated air at work—all of which has left your body, and most of its systems, dry and parched. Unless you've been supplying water throughout the day, dehydration is your problem.

If you are attuned and sensitive enough to your body's signals, you should be able to recognize some of the early warnings of dehydration:

- Dizziness
- Headache
- Fatigue
- Thirst
- Flushed skin
- Blurred vision
- Muscle weakness

These warning signs merit your attention. Unfortunately, most people never realize that they spend most days in a state of partial dehydration.

Although thirst is an important warning sign, many people seem to be desensitized to the signal. Some people, especially adults over forty, may actually have a decreased sensation of thirst.

Water and Fat Loss

Invariably the individuals in my fat-loss programs who consistently drink the most water, consistently lose the most fat. Here's why plenty of water worked for them, and why it will work for you:

Kidney-liver function. Your kidneys require abundant water to function properly. If your kidneys do not get enough water, your liver takes over and assumes some of the functions of the kidneys. This diverts your liver from its primary duty—to metabolize stored fat into usable energy.

If your liver is preoccupied with performing the chores of your water-depleted kidneys, it doesn't efficiently convert the stored materials into usable chemicals. Thus, your fat loss stops, or it at least plateaus. Superhydration actually accelerates your fat-loss process.

Appetite control. Lots of water flowing over your tongue keeps your taste buds cleansed of flavors that might otherwise trigger a craving. Furthermore, water keeps your stomach feeling full between meals, which can help take the edge off your appetite.

"I used to suffer from what I thought was a raging appetite," remembers one of the middle-aged men who lost thirty pounds on the ASAP plan, "but

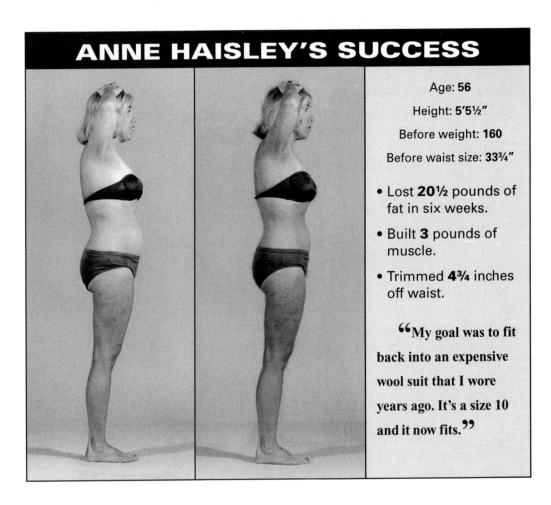

ANNE HAISLEY'S SUCCESS

Age: **56**

Height: **5'5½"**

Before weight: **160**

Before waist size: **33¾"**

- Lost **20½** pounds of fat in six weeks.
- Built **3** pounds of muscle.
- Trimmed **4¾** inches off waist.

"My goal was to fit back into an expensive wool suit that I wore years ago. It's a size 10 and it now fits."

eating never seemed to satisfy me very long. Now, I know that what I was really suffering from was simple dehydration. Once my dehydration was cured, my raging appetite vanished."

Urine production. Remember in chapter 2, when I pointed out that as much as 85 percent of your daily heat loss emerged through your skin? That means the remaining 15 percent of your daily heat loss must leave from somewhere else. And it does: through your lungs and through your urine. Although you lose a small amount of heat through your feces, it's not significant unless you suffer from diarrhea. If you're typical, approximately 10 percent of your daily calories and heat loss goes through your lungs, and 5 percent leaves through your urine. But what if you could double, triple, or even quadruple your urine production? Would that be helpful? Yes, and you can with the ASAP superhydration plan.

Most adults in the United States drink no more than the traditionally recommended six to eight glasses of water a day. Many people don't even get that much. No wonder Americans are the fattest people on earth. Certainly, there are many other reasons involved in why Americans are so fat, but the fact that most Americans do not have consistent water-drinking habits is a neglected consideration that needs much discussion.

Think back for a minute to our Ice Age ancestors. Doesn't it make sense that even mild dehydration was a strong warning signal that something was wrong? And when something was wrong, our Ice Age ancestors' bodies went into a survival mode that preserved fat. My research shows that our modern bodies do the same thing. Lack of water tells your body to preserve fat. Gradually increasing your consumption of water encourages your body to give up its fat freely.

That's exactly what you'll be doing on the ASAP superhydration plan. You'll be drinking from 1 to 1¾ gallons of water each day. The specifics of how to do this will be detailed in chapter 9. In case you're wondering how your body holds all that water, it does so remarkably well and even thrives on it. Remember, your body is composed of up to 65 percent water.

As your body gradually becomes superhydrated, it steps up the production of urine—which it must do to allow you to lose heat calories or fat in the fastest, most efficient way. So get used to going to the bathroom regularly.

Cold-water connection. Have you ever wished for a food that contains negative calories? For discussion purposes, let's say such a food exists and it contains minus a hundred calories per serving. Anytime you feel like a candy bar, a piece of chocolate cake, or a donut, all you have to do is simply follow the sweet snack with several servings of the negative-calorie food. Presto—plus two hundred calories and minus two hundred calories yields zero calories. While no negative-caloric food exists, at least not yet in the world of science, ice-cold water can have a similar effect inside your body.

When you drink ice water, which is about 40 degrees Fahrenheit, your system has to heat the fluid to a core body temperature of 98.6 degrees. This process requires almost one calorie to warm one ounce of cold water to body temperature. Thus, an eight-ounce glass of ice water burns approximately 8 calories, or 7.69 calories to be exact. Extend that over sixteen glasses, 128 ounces, or one gallon—and you've generated 123 calories of heat energy, which is significant. A professor of biology from the University of Florida, who superhydrated through the ASAP program, added to my understanding of the cold-water connection when he pointed out that melting ice and a burning candle both require the transfer of heat. They simply modify their forms. The ice changes from solid to liquid, and the candle from solid to gas. Both transfers or changes involve heat.

Constipation help. When deprived of water, your system pulls cellular fluid from your lower intestines and bowel, creating hard, dry stools. One of the big roles of water is to flush waste from the body. This is a substantial task during fat metabolism because waste tends to accumulate quickly. Thus, superhydration tends to make people more regular and consistent with their bowel movements, which is helpful to the overall fat-loss process.

Tap Water Concerns

Many people are concerned about the safety of drinking water from the tap. How safe your tap water is depends on where you live. Statistics from the Environmental Protection Agency, the government service charged with insuring safe drinking water, suggest that approximately 20 percent of the community water supplies in the United States do not meet safety standards. Tap water can be contaminated with bacteria, metals, radon, and a host of many other chemicals and pollutants.

The government requires that your community's water plant test regularly for contaminants. You can get the latest results of this testing by phoning your local water department. If you are seriously concerned after examining the report, you can then contact the Environmental Protection Agency's Safe Drinking Water Hotline (800-426-4791) to pursue the matter further. You'll find this hotline very helpful.

Chances are, however, that your local water supply is reasonably safe. But you can certainly relieve some of your concern about safety with the installation of a filter on your faucet. These filtering systems cost from $30 to more than $500. And price is not a sure indicator of quality. Before you purchase one, check with the manufacturer to see if it has been tested by the Environmental Protection Agency.

Bottled Water

Bottled water has turned into a multibillion-dollar business in the United States. Something like 15 percent of our population regularly drink bottled water, with those living in California heading the list. Interestingly, bottled water has to meet fewer safety standards for contaminants than tap water. Research around the country shows that bottled water is not always of higher quality than tap water. The decision to drink bottled water or not is usually one of taste.

If you dislike the taste of your tap water, then drink your favorite bottled water. If you have no problems with your local water, then save some money and consume it.

Water Versus Other Beverages

Here's a statistic that will surprise you. The average American in 1990 drank forty-two gallons of soda (regular and diet) and only forty-one gallons of tap water. Obviously those of us involved with superhydration hope to change that statistic.

But does it really make a difference whether you drink water, sodas, or other beverages as long as you get the required fluids into your system? Yes, it does make a difference because other drinks have substances that may contradict some of the positive benefits of the extra water.

Sodas, soft drinks, coffee, and tea contain caffeine, which stimulates the adrenal glands and acts as a diuretic. Some beverages are loaded with calories from sugar and alcohol. In addition, drinking too many flavored beverages can decrease your taste for water.

Speaking of caffeine and alcohol, I'd prefer that you give up beverages that contain them for the duration of the ASAP program; you'll get more efficient results if you do.

The way to interpret all of this is that your recommended daily water intake means just that—water. Even people who heighten the taste of their water with a twist of lemon or lime eventually get to the point where they prefer their water with nothing added.

Too Much Water

Yes, it's possible to drink too much water—but it's highly unlikely that you would ever do so. In the medical literature, drinking too much water leads to a condition known as hyponatremia.

I've read about hyponatremia occurring in a few athletes involved in triathlons and ultramarathons. The athletes consume many gallons of water during the course of these unusually long competitions, and because of the continuous activity they don't or can't stop to urinate. Thus, they impede their normal fluid-mineral balance and actually become intoxicated with too much water. Such a condition, however, is extremely rare.

I've never observed anything close to intoxication happening with any of my participants, and many of them consume two gallons of water daily. Of course, they also have no trouble urinating frequently.

Note: Anyone with a kidney disorder or anyone who takes diuretics should consult a physician before making any modifications of his or her water consumption.

Attack . . . Copy . . . Steal

While a few experts and advisors are busy trying to ignore, ridicule, and attack my views and recommendations on superhydration, you've had a chance to examine and understand the facts. Water is an essential key to health. Most people simply don't drink enough of it.

It's now time for you to apply the guidelines and start reaping the benefits. Superhydration has worked for thousands of people. It will work for you.

When it does, I want you to spread the idea.

Copy it.

Steal it.

Call it your own. But get the message out. People need superhydration.

Let's drink to it.

On the rocks and straight up—WATER!

7

SLEEP:

RELIEVE THE STRESS

A five-dollar bet. That was what I made with Lydia Maree, my favorite instructor who helps me with the ASAP strength-training programs at the Gainesville Health & Fitness Center.

I usually bet her that during the introduction/sign-up meetings, I can correctly guess the woman and man who will lose the most fat over the next six weeks.

During the meeting in June of 1996, it was obvious to me that the couple seated in the front row would do the best. They were attentive, pleasantly plump, and both tall. Most of all, however, they had a certain look that let me know that they were very serious about this endeavor. Their names were Paige and Jeffrey Arnold.

After the meeting, I told Lydia of my choices. Lydia, being biased for short women and men, disagreed with me. Thus the bet was established.

Jeff began the program with a bang. Just as I had predicted, his body weight dropped in a steady stair-stepped fashion—from 219 to 215 to 211 to 208 to 204. At the end of the first two weeks, Jeff had lost fifteen pounds.

Paige, on the other hand, was a different story. Her every-other-day body weight readings were as follows: 150, 153, 152, 150, 150. Her weight went up slightly and then came back down. In two weeks, she had not lost a single pound.

You can imagine how she felt. She and her husband are both on the same basic program. He drops fifteen pounds and she loses zero pounds.

What was wrong?

After talking with Paige, I realized she was not getting enough sleep. Paige worked at a radio station in Gainesville and had to get up most mornings at 4:00 A.M. Most nights, she was lucky to sleep for five hours. Furthermore, she had a lot of job-related stress that was affecting her in significant ways.

Lack of sleep and too much stress can curb even the best fat-loss program, or at least slow it down to a mere trickle. I've found that the most fat loss occurs when you get not just a normal amount of sleep but also more sleep than what you normally get.

Extra sleep is necessary if you're dieting and strength training. Efficient fat loss and muscle building both require a rested recovery ability.

Recovery Ability

Recovery ability involves the chemical reactions that are necessary for your body to overcompensate and get leaner and stronger. An optimum recovery ability is dependent primarily on adequate rest and sufficient time.

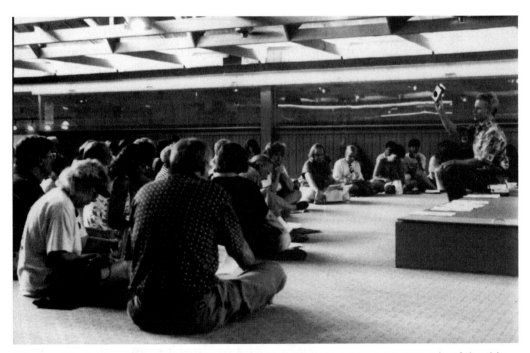

Ellington Darden, seated on the riser at the right, displays to a group an example of the thin-sliced turkey breast that he recommends as a lunch selection. During these introductory meetings Dr. Darden sizes up the new ASAP participants.

Your body is a complex factory that is constantly making hundreds of delicate changes to transform food and oxygen into many chemicals required by various parts of the system. But there is a limit to the chemical conversions that your recovery ability can make within a given time. If your requirements exceed the limit, your body will eventually be overworked to the point of collapse.

Years ago, researchers focused on sleep as a brain phenomenon, ignoring the other parts of the body. Now they recognize that sleep regulates body temperature, replenishes the immune system, and yields hormones that facilitate fat loss and strength building.

How much sleep is enough? To answer this question, let's explore the sleep cycle.

The Sleep Cycle

An infant sleeps 14 hours a day, a typical adult averages 7½ hours, and people over seventy-five years old manage only 6 hours. New studies reveal that the length of sleep is not what causes you to be refreshed as much as it is the number of sleep cycles you complete. For practical purposes, it is sufficient to say that one sleep cycle lasts an average of ninety minutes. This ninety minutes is composed of sixty-five minutes of normal sleep, twenty minutes of rapid-eye-movement sleep (in which you dream), and a final five minutes of normal sleep. The middle, rapid-eye-movement phase tends to be shorter during earlier cycles and longer during later ones. But still, each of these cycles tends to remain constant at ninety minutes or 1½ hours.

If you closely monitor your natural sleeping patterns, you will wake up, on the average, after multiples of 1½ hours. In other words, you will wake up after 4½ hours, 6 hours, 7½ hours, or 9 hours—but not after 7 or 8 hours, since these numbers are not multiples of 1½ hours. In the period between cycles you are not actually sleeping. It is a sort of twilight zone from which, if you are not disturbed, you progress into another 1½-hour cycle.

Interestingly, a person who sleeps only four cycles or six hours will feel more rested than someone who has slept for eight to ten hours but has not been allowed to finish any one cycle because of being awakened before it was completed.

Thus it's important that you try to better plan your sleeping around multiples of these 1½-hour cycles. Most of you are probably getting too little sleep for maximum fat loss and strength building. Most of you could profit by adding at least one more ninety-minute cycle to your sleep each night.

Naps

A nap, unlike a ninety-minute sleep cycle, is simply a brief rest period that involves closing your eyes and relaxing. You may or may not lie in a bed to take a nap. Some people practice naps and meditations seated in a chair to achieve the same benefits.

The ideal time to take a nap seems to be between noon and 3:00 P.M., and the ideal length seems to be fifteen to thirty minutes. The worst time to nap is early evening, as this could interfere with your nightly sleep cycles.

A nap at the right time can definitely help you to recover and mobilize fat cells into action as you recharge for the remainder of the day.

Your Bed

Since you will spend about one-third of your life in bed, it's important to examine this important piece of furniture.

To allow restful sleep, your bed should be:

Big. You should be able to roll over multiple times each night without disturbing your sleep or your partner. A sixty-inch-wide bed (queen size) is adequate for two normal sleepers. But if you or your partner is a restless sleeper, a seventy-two-inch wide bed (king size) may be more appropriate.

Comfortable. Comfort from your point of view may come from a hard, medium, or soft spring mattress, air mattress, or cotton-stuffed futon. Or it could involve rubber sponge, plastic sponge, or the gentle waves of a water bed. There's a fiercely competitive market today where mattresses and beds are concerned. You should take considerable time in checking them out.

Dry. Your bed's sheets, covers, and pillows also should be selected carefully. High-quality cotton sheets can be purchased that feel like fine silk in the spring and toasty flannel in the fall. A wide variety of covers and pillows is also available. Give them all a try before you decide. But whatever you finally choose, make sure you keep your bed dry and well aired.

Humans, as you should know by now, are surprisingly damp creatures—and superhydration will add more fluids to your skin. As a result, you'll probably perspire at least a pint of sweat into your bedding each night. Thus it's a good idea to make sure your mattress receives proper airing. Most beds provide some way to let air get at the underside of the mattress. This is the main reason why it is not a good idea to sleep on the floor. The bedding does not get aired properly. Ten minutes with the covers pulled back to the foot of the bed in a breezy or warm room will take the moisture out. Also make sure you launder your sheets at least once a week.

Your Bedroom

Your bedroom also merits equal attention. Here are some things you can do to turn this area into a superb sleep room.

Take a close look at your bedroom. What potential sleep-disturbing objects do you see? Is there a television available? Are there magazines and newspapers on your night table or floor? Is there a telephone a few feet from your bed? Is a work desk or sewing table part of the furniture? Each of these items could impede your sleep. Maybe you'd be better off if you relocated some or all of these items to other, less serious rooms in your house. Doing so would certainly change the mood in your bedroom.

To get the best sleep, your bedroom should be:

Dark. Darkness has a natural and healthy connection to sleep. Humans are creatures of the day, and the sleep we need is linked to the dark. Light is therefore a deterrent to sleep. Think about light pollution when choosing your house, apartment, or picking your sleep room. Blinds or curtains can help keep out sunlight as well as city lights, but aluminum foil taped to your bedroom windows can provide almost total darkness and will help keep your area cool.

Ventilated. Two people, after sleeping for four hours in a ten-by-thirteen feet bedroom with no ventilation will be breathing air that is 15 percent stale. Breathing stale air is no way to sleep well, so it's important to ventilate your bedroom. If opening a window lets in noise, an open window in a nearby bathroom or other room can bring you fresh air. Fans can also circulate air throughout your sleep room.

Quiet. Loud music playing in the apartment above yours, a barking dog next door, or a motorcycle gunning its way on the street below can make it difficult to fall asleep. Sure, some people claim to be able to sleep through even the worst thunderstorm, but the vast majority of sleepers can be aroused by even the sounds of air conditioners down the hall and refrigeration two rooms away. Even if such a noise doesn't awaken you, it still takes its toll and lowers the quality of your sleep. Do your best to tame these outside noises.

A prevalent sound in your bedroom may be your clock. A high-quality digital clock will solve that problem.

And let's not forget about the telephone, which can be the most common noisemaker of all. Put an answering machine on your telephone and remove the extension entirely from your bedroom—or at the very least do so on those occasions when sleep is a must. Do not be a slave to your telephone.

Security and Safety

Your sleep room should be a refuge where you can escape from the world. This means locking the door to keep people out. It also means taking steps to safeguard against smoke and fire.

In your home you will probably leave your bedroom unlocked and depend on your front door to provide security. Make sure you have the necessary bolts, chains, and alarms to discourage and keep out intruders. A simple lock on your bedroom door can supply additional security as well as privacy.

In many apartments, the door to your sleep room is your front door. Check with the management about the existing locks and keys. They may need to be changed, depending on who the last tenants were. Also, inquire about night security people who patrol the area, and keep track of their schedules.

Equally important is to do a thorough check of all fire hazards in your home or apartment. Correct anything that looks suspicious. Install and maintain smoke detectors. Keep a fire extinguisher handy and in plain sight.

Peace of mind and a good night's sleep come from knowing that your home and bedroom are secure and safe.

Sleep Cooler

Remember from the chapter on superhydration when I explained how your body has to warm cold water that you drink? Warming cold water requires heat calories, and that's good from the standpoint of losing fat. Your body will also require additional heat calories if you learn to sleep slightly cooler than you normally do. I'm convinced that too many people bury themselves under too many covers when they sleep.

Your body requires at least fifty calories per hour while sleeping to keep it functioning normally. Thus, a typical night of sleep burns four hundred calories, most of which goes to keeping your body warm. But by learning to sleep a little cooler, you can force your body to turn up its thermostat and burn more fat to keep you warm. Though doing this may be a little uncomfortable for a while, it can be mastered.

If you tend to sleep under thick covers, try to eliminate one or two layers. Wean yourself from using an electric blanket and flannel sheets during the winter months. In summer, pull only a sheet over you. Then experiment with one leg on top of the sheet. You'll be amazed at how easily your body adapts.

It won't be long until you'll be generating an extra ten to twenty calories per hour while you sleep.

Sleep and Stress

There seems to be a definite relationship between a lack of sleep and too much stress in a person's life. Getting better quality sleep tends to help a person cope more with stress, and dealing with stress productively tends to allow a person to sleep better.

This was certainly the case with Paige Arnold, whom I introduced at the beginning of this chapter. As Paige began to get more sleep, she found that she could more effectively deal with her job stress. To her delight, her body weight started to drop. At the end of the fourth week, she had gone from 150 to 143, for a loss of seven pounds.

Jeff, who started with a bang, continued with his steady decline in body fat. By the end of the fourth week, he had lost twenty-five pounds and all his pants were bagging around his waist. Of course, Jeff had no trouble sleeping and no stress in his life that he couldn't deal with. Or as Paige said, "Jeff's about as easygoing and not affected by stress as anybody can be. It's just not fair, is it?"

Excessive Stress

Whether it's fair or not, too much stress can provide major hurdles as you progress through the fat-loss process. Below is a listing of physical stresses that can cause your body to hold on to fat:

- *A very low-calorie diet:* under 1,200 calories a day for men and 1,000 calories a day for women.
- *Too little dietary fat:* less than thirty grams a day for men and twenty grams a day for women.
- *Too much strength training or other types of exercise:* longer than forty-five minutes per workout, or more frequently than three times per week.
- *Too little sleep:* less than six hours sleep per night.
- *Dehydration:* A loss of one percent of the body's water can cause alarm.
- *Excessive heat:* High levels of environmental heat can reduce the body's efficiency.

- *Accumulated problems* about work or relationships can also have negative effects.
- *Sicknesses, drugs, or extreme behaviors* can send survival signals to the body.

Instead of stressed-out actions, you want to communicate to your body that everything is well. You do this best by avoiding extremes and by practicing moderation, moderation in almost everything—except your strength training. Moderately hard strength training is not very productive. Strength training that is performed in the super-slow style is extremely intense—as it must be—to achieve the fastest possible, muscular growth stimulation.

How does muscular growth stimulation send a positive message to your body to part with its fat? Once again, we must look back to our ancient ancestors for the answer.

Muscular Strength and Survival

One of the fundamental necessities of our Ice Age ancestors' lives was locomotion or movement. Movement depended on muscular strength. Anthropological research shows that survival resources were allocated to the muscles first. An individual had to be able to run fast and fight fiercely to eat and avoid being eaten. In other words, hard, brief activity produced stronger muscles, and stronger muscles led to success at hunting and in battle. Stronger, larger muscles improved the probability of survival.

Today, when you go on an even moderately reduced-calorie diet, your body perceives that something is wrong. It kicks into its survival mechanism, which prevents you from losing fat in the most efficient manner.

To prevent this from occurring, you have to override your long-term survival mechanisms by stimulating your muscles to grow with proper strength training. Your growing muscles will then draw calories from your fat cells. Doing so significantly increases the effectiveness and efficiency of your ability to reduce fat. Doing so makes you leaner and stronger faster.

Back to Paige and Jeff

Paige Arnold, after a slow start on the ASAP course, rebounded by losing 7 pounds during the middle two weeks and another 7½ pounds over the last two weeks. In total, she lost 14½ pounds of fat—all of which was accomplished in the last four weeks. Even more impressive was the fact that Paige built 6 pounds of muscle. She would have probably done even better on both her muscle building and fat loss if she had started the course with better sleeping habits.

In spite of her lack of initial progress, Paige still finished second in total fat loss among the women in her group. But second place is not the same as first, and I had to pay five dollars to Lydia. Actually, the five dollars was canceled out because I did guess correctly for the men's group by picking Jeff Arnold.

Jeff completed *A Flat Stomach ASAP* by dropping 33¾ pounds of fat and 5¼ inches from his waist.

Both Jeff and Paige, while being pleased with their results, still felt they had some more fat to remove. I agreed. Thus they immediately decided to continue the plan for another six weeks using the guidelines described in chapter 13.

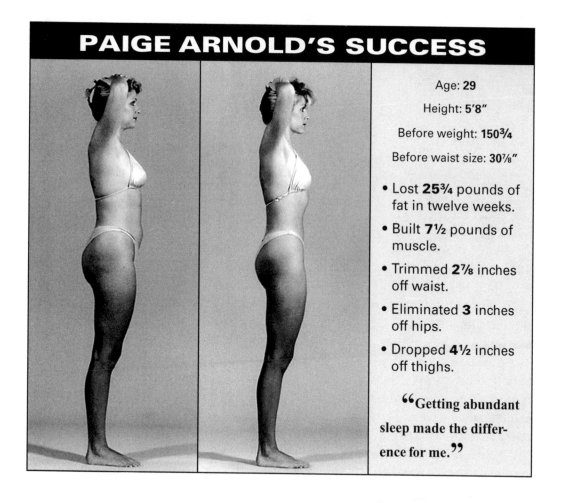

PAIGE ARNOLD'S SUCCESS

Age: **29**

Height: **5'8"**

Before weight: **150¾**

Before waist size: **30⅞"**

- Lost **25¾** pounds of fat in twelve weeks.
- Built **7½** pounds of muscle.
- Trimmed **2⅞** inches off waist.
- Eliminated **3** inches off hips.
- Dropped **4½** inches off thighs.

❝Getting abundant sleep made the difference for me.❞

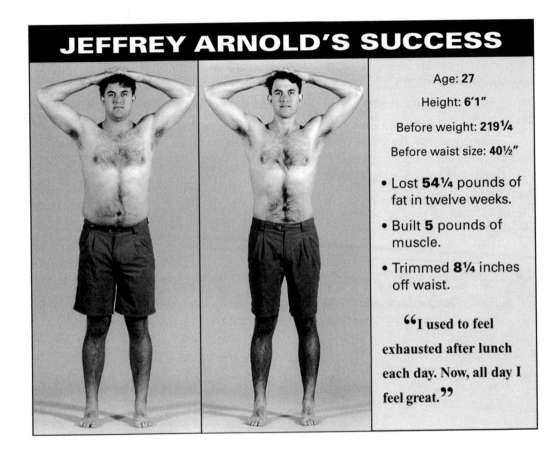

JEFFREY ARNOLD'S SUCCESS

Age: **27**

Height: **6'1"**

Before weight: **219¼**

Before waist size: **40½"**

- Lost **54¼** pounds of fat in twelve weeks.
- Built **5** pounds of muscle.
- Trimmed **8¼** inches off waist.

"I used to feel exhausted after lunch each day. Now, all day I feel great."

After another six weeks, their overall results were dramatic. Paige lost 11¼ more pounds for a grand total of 25¾ pounds of fat. Jeff shed an additional 20½ pounds for a combined total of 54¼ pounds. Jeff's waist shrank by 8¼ inches, a remarkable drop. At the start, Paige's belly didn't bulge to the same degree that Jeff's did. Her fat was stored more over her hips and thighs. Thus, she lost 3 inches off her hips and 4½ inches off her thighs.

"Some of our friends and relatives who hadn't seen Jeff and me in six months saw us over the Christmas holidays," Paige recently noted. "A few just stared. Others wanted to know exactly what we had done. My mother-in-law, who usually gives me clothes, noted that this year's sweater was four sizes smaller than last year's.

"And Jeffrey, well he's been on cloud nine from all the attention he's gotten. Ever since I met Jeff, he's been a sharp dresser. Even though he bought all these Italian-style clothes, he could never quite pull it off with that forty-inch waist. Now, it's different.

"Those broad shoulders and that tiny waist tucked into his new Armani suit—wow! When I hug him now, it's like having a whole new husband."

Paige, by the way, recently released her first singing album, which is called *You Knew Me When*. If everything goes as expected, she'll soon be in demand.

Contratulations are in order for Paige and Jeff.

Sounds like they'll both be able, in the future, to sleep well.

Furthermore, all the mechanics should be falling in place for you to do the same.

8

Synergy:

Maximize the Process

I
t seems impossible, according to the scientific literature, to lose fat as rapidly as do the participants in my ASAP program.

The average fat loss for a man is 3.83 pounds per week, or 23 pounds in six weeks. For a woman, the figures are 2.5 pounds per week and 15 pounds in six weeks. Realize, too, that these are *averages*. Some of my people, as you no doubt have noticed from the success stories throughout this book, drop significantly more pounds of fat.

Many scientists presume such weight losses are helped by dehydration— until they find out that my course accentuates the opposite: superhydration. Other scientists note that my figures are higher because my trainees are also losing muscle—until they learn that I perform skin fold measurements and strength tests on my subjects. My trainees actually build muscle, not lose it.

Strength training and superhydrating, combined with reduced-calorie eating, are big reasons for the success of *A Flat Stomach ASAP*. But another reason, and one that most scientists don't account for—is *synergy*, which is where several factors interact to yield greater return than the sum of the parts.

In other words, if strength training, superhydrating, and reduced-calorie eating *each* produce one-half pound of fat loss per week, then the expected sum should be 1½ pounds. Except it isn't. As a result of synergy, it yields 3, or even 3½ pounds of fat loss.

Recognizing the effect is not as meaningful as determining why and how synergy works.

Unraveling Synergy

Humans are heat-producing mammals governed by thermodynamics. Our bodies produce and transfer hundreds and hundreds of calories of heat energy each day. Most of this heat energy keeps our bodies warm and at equilibrium.

As stated previously, body fat is best expressed as calories—or units of heat energy. One pound of fat equals 3,500 calories.

Your body gets rid of fat calories or heat in three ways: through your kidneys, lungs, and skin.

Superhydration has a triple fat-burning effect on your system. First, it increases urination. Second, your body requires 123 calories of energy to heat one gallon of 40-degree Fahrenheit fluid to the 98.6-degree Fahrenheit temperature

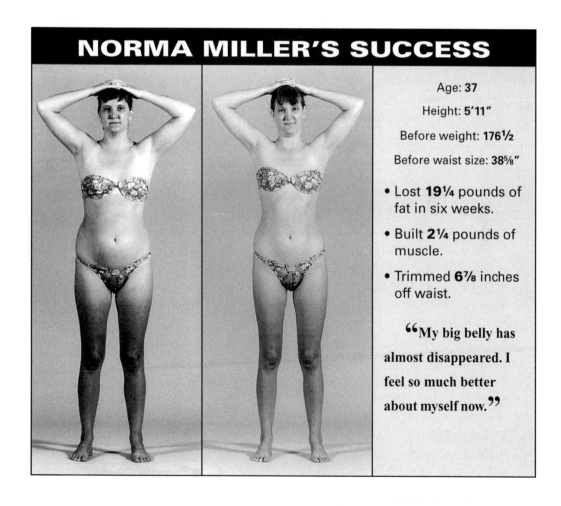

NORMA MILLER'S SUCCESS

Age: **37**

Height: **5′11″**

Before weight: **176½**

Before waist size: **38⅝″**

- Lost **19¼** pounds of fat in six weeks.
- Built **2¼** pounds of muscle.
- Trimmed **6⅞** inches off waist.

❝My big belly has almost disappeared. I feel so much better about myself now.❞

of your urinary system. Third, your liver functions more efficiently if it has large volumes of water when mobilizing fat. At least 15 percent of your daily heat loss is a result of superhydration's impact on your kidneys.

Another 10 percent of your heat transfer goes through your lungs. Your lungs act as a bellows. Inhalation brings in oxygen-rich air, which is vital for energy metabolism. Exhalation carries out oxygen-poor air and carbon dioxide—which both exist as warm gases.

The remaining 75 percent of your daily heat calories is eliminated through your skin. A tall, lean person has a larger skin surface area than another person who is the same weight but shorter and stockier. Because the tall person constantly loses more calories by radiation, he can consume more calories than the shorter person. Radiant heat is why shorter people, who emit less of it, tend to get heavier and taller people, who emit more of it, tend to remain lean.

Your skin also eliminates significant heat by conduction, the transfer of calories through direct contant. Conduction is the primary reason that ice-cold fluid inside the body generates significant heat. It's why an almost-shivering state mobilizes three times as many calories as sweating.

Thermodynamic Tips

The science behind thermodynamics is why I want you to practice the following:

- Try to remain uncomfortably cool throughout the day and allow your skin's heating mechanism to adjust.
- Make sure your drinking water is chilled.
- Dress cooler and lighter at work.
- Take off your coat sooner and keep it off longer.
- Select short sleeves more often.
- Don't wear a hat.
- Turn down the thermostat.
- Strength train in a cooler environment if possible.
- Wear brief, well-ventilated clothing when you train.
- Minimize sweating by eliminating heat buildup.
- Shun sauna, steam, and whirlpool baths, as they cause excessive heat accumulation.
- Sleep cooler.
- Wean yourself from electric blankets and flannel sheets in the winter.
- Experiment with having one leg on top of the sheet during the summer.

Strength Training and Metabolism

Besides making you look, feel, and perform better, strength training speeds up your metabolism. Remember, other than your brain and internal organs, it's your skeletal muscles that have the most energy potential.

Add a pound of muscle to your body through proper strength training and your metabolism goes up approximately 37.5 calories per day. Interestingly, the average person who progresses through *A Flat Stomach ASAP* adds at least 3½ pounds of muscle to his or her body. Three and one-half pounds of muscle means that individual will burn 131.25 more calories per day.

Recall also that fat influences metabolism. Each pound needs approximately 2 calories a day to keep alive. Muscle, by comparison, is 18.75 times more energy demanding than the same amount of fat.

Obviously, losing fat without building muscle is not a good idea. Doing so simply lowers metabolism. But adding as little as one pound of muscle would compensate for the metabolic loss of almost nineteen pounds of fat. Even better is to build as much muscle as you can—four, five, or possibly six pounds—in the six-week course.

Larger, stronger muscles are true synergy in action.

Other Synergistic Dynamics

There are other practices that contribute synergistically to fat loss. You should consider each one:

Find a friend to go through the ASAP program with you. You'll probably get better fat-loss and strength-training results if you go through the course with a friend. Both you and your friend should be serious about making a six-week commitment. That commitment means you'll be exercising together three times a week, talking on the phone often, shopping together, monitoring each other's water intake, and sharing problems.

Walk moderately after your evening meal. If you walk at a leisurely pace for thirty minutes with food and cold water in your belly, you'll speed up your body's ability to release heat calories. Begin your walks within fifteen minutes after you finish your meal. Your goal is to cover no more than 1½ to 2 miles. Wear well-constructed and comfortable walking or running shoes. Walk outdoors, if possible, on level ground. Or you may substitute a bicycle ride for the walk. If the weather is a problem, you may walk indoors or use a stationary bicycle or a treadmill.

Reduce salt (sodium) intake. The average adult in the United States consumes three or four times more salt or sodium each day than required. Aside from the relationship between excessive sodium and high-blood pressure, and excessive sodium and fluid retention, salt generally hangs out with high-calorie foods. There seems to be an almost irresistible urge to eat foods that contain salt, fat, and sugar. And one you start, it's difficult to stop. All the recommended foods on the ASAP eating plan are low in salt. None of your daily menus contains more than 2,400 milligrams of sodium. You can do your part by hiding your salt shaker. You won't need it for the duration of this course.

Learn and practice doing a stomach vacuum. Here's a trick I learned years ago from a champion bodybuilder. During his onstage posing routine, this body-

The stomach vacuum, correctly applied, exerts a concave action on the transverse abdominis muscles.

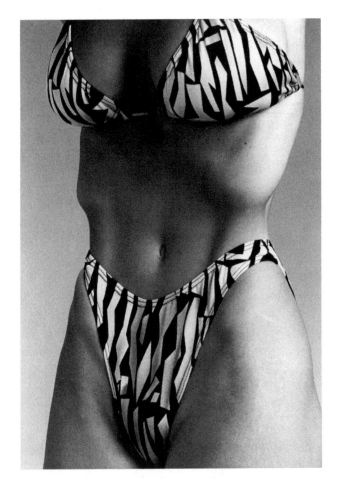

builder could suddenly suck in his stomach to such a degree that you could almost see his backbone from the front. Then he would proceed to pop out his cleanly defined abdominal muscles one at a time from top to bottom. It was an impressive display of muscle control and contributed greatly to this man's winning many physique contests.

It's the first part of this trick, the sucking in of the stomach, that I want to teach you. It involves an unusual contraction of your transverse abdominis, the deep horizontal muscle that stretches across your middle. I taught this contraction to a hundred women who went through one of my tummy-tightening courses, and most of them got the hang of it quickly.

To practice a vacuum, you must have a relatively empty stomach. Here's what to do:

- Lie in bed on your back.
- Place your hands across the bottom of your rib cage and top of your abdominals.
- Take a normal breath and forcibly blow out as much air as possible. This should require about ten seconds.
- Suck in your stomach to the maximum degree. It's important, however, that you take in no air during this process. You should feel a concave formation under your rib cage. You won't be able to hold this vacuum feat very long.
- Try the vacuum several more times while lying down. If you feel a little light-headed, that's normal. Rest a bit longer between trials.
- Stand now and get in front of a mirror and try the vacuum. Remove your shirt so you can see what's happening. At first, the vacuum is more difficult to do standing than lying, but with a little more practice, you should be able to master it in a standing position.
- Practice the stomach vacuum twice before breakfast, lunch, and dinner—or six times a day—for two weeks. After two weeks, you should have mastered the contraction of your transverse abdominis muscles—and as a result they'll be significantly stronger.
- Continue to apply the stomach vacuum six times a day for the duration of the ASAP course, and the involved muscles will become even stronger and more under your control.

Avoid doing strenuous activities or other exercises on the days you do not strength train. Too much activity can be more harmful than too little activity, especially when you're following a reduced-calorie diet. If you strength train intensely more than three times per week, your system soon reaches a state of overtraining. Fat losses and strength gains slow rather than accelerate. At this point you are close to *burning the candle at both ends* and trying to light it in the middle too.

During your participation in the ASAP course, it's to your advantage to keep your outside activities to a minimum. Naturally, you can continue with your normal work and household responsibilities. Simply avoid rigorous activities such as running, aerobics classes, skiing, racquetball, and basketball. Light recreational games not carried to extremes are probably fine, but if in doubt, don't do them. Once you reach your fat-loss goal, you can get involved in various strenuous sports and fitness activities if you wish.

Use color wisely. Intense color can stimulate your appetite. Don't use place settings or tablecloths of warm red, bright yellow, lime green, or orange. Even worse may be the red-and-white checkered tablecloths you often see in Italian restaurants and pizza parlors. You'll eat less on white or pale plates and tablecloths.

Watch only essential television programs. TV exposes you to multimillion-dollar advertisements that know how to prompt you to buy and to eat. Such advertising has its fingers on all our impulse buttons. Make it a personal rule never to eat while watching TV. Limit your exposure by selecting TV viewing that is essential. Getting outside for a walk and going to bed earlier than normal will help you break the evening TV habit.

Begin a household project. To take your mind off food and keep your hands busy, start a major project around the house. How about wallpapering the kitchen, painting the garage, or refinishing a table? Any number of other undertakings would be just as good. Get involved at home and stay active.

Incorporate good posture. Proper posture burns more calories than does poor posture. Correct stature automatically forces you to tighten your abdominal muscles. The best posture resembles a marionette with a string attached to the top of the head. Imagine being tugged gently upward by the string.

I recommend that the ASAP participants not only visualize the string pulling up but also focus on keeping the top of their heads forced up toward the ceiling. This recommendation applies well to sitting, standing, and walking. Furthermore, these practices project greater height which, by itself, emphasizes thinness.

Brush your teeth often. The next time you're really hungry, brush your teeth and use a tingly, minty toothpaste. During the process, also brush your tongue. Afterward, you'll find that it's more difficult to consume rich foods with intense flavors. Sweets, for example, tend to taste bitter temporarily after certain tingly toothpastes have been used. This may be just the reminder you need to skip a rich appetizer, tempting dessert, or sugary snack.

Be proactive. Direct your eating behaviors around your own conscious choices, which are based on tried-and-proved guidelines, as opposed to making reactive choices, which flow from physical and social environments.

With the ASAP course, as you become leaner and stronger, you will automatically become more proactive and more assertive. Soon, you'll be saying *No!* to certain foods and temptations, and *Yes!* to things that are beneficial to your health and fitness. It won't be long before you'll be in control—in *complete* control of your life.

APPLICATION

Part Three

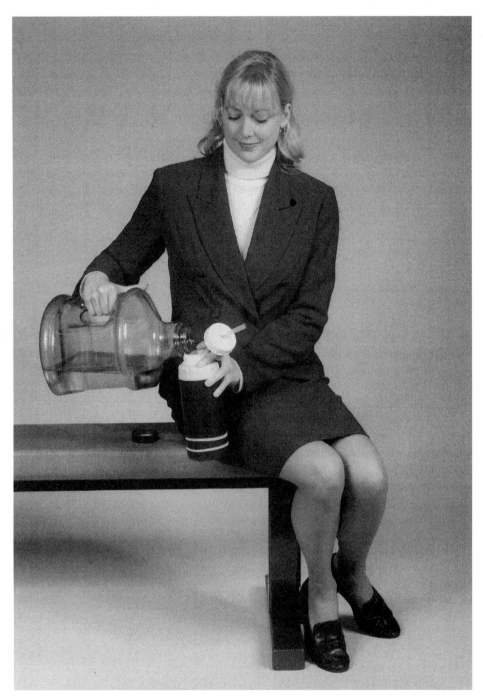

To help you track your daily water consumption, this picture illustrates four efficient guidelines. First, the clear plastic jug holds two gallons, which serves as a one-day reservoir for your water. Second, the water is being poured into a thirty-two-ounce, insulated bottle that keeps your water chilled. Third, the top contains a plastic straw for easy sipping. Fourth, the rubber bands around the bottom let you know how many more bottles you have to drink to meet your quota.

9

ATTENTION:

INITIATE IMPORTANT STEPS

There are a number of important steps and guidelines to initiate before starting *A Flat Stomach ASAP*. Devoting the necessary attention to each step will make it easier for you to accomplish your goals.

Check with Your Physician

Your doctor should be aware that you are about to modify your eating and physical fitness habits. Take this book with you for easy referral. Your physician will more than likely recommend a thorough physical examination if you have not had one in the last twelve months.

There are a few people who should not try this program: children and teenagers; pregnant women; women who are breast-feeding; men and women with certain types of heart, liver, or kidney disease; diabetics; and those suffering from some types of arthritis and cancer. This should not be taken as an all-inclusive list. Some individuals should follow the ASAP course only with their physician's specific guidance. Consult your health care professional beforehand and play it safe.

Do Your Measurements and Photographs

Don't procrastinate on taking your measurements and photographs. Without accurate assessments, you'll be traveling a difficult road without a good support system. Get out your bathing suit, tape measure, and camera—turn back to chapter 3 for a quick review—and proceed one step at a time.

Buy Food Measuring Spoons, Cups, and a Small Scale

Most people have a tendency to overestimate one ounce of cheese, two ounces of turkey, or four ounces of skim milk. Such practices lead to inaccurate calorie counting and inefficient fat reduction. It's important to become familiar with and correctly use measuring spoons, cups, and food scales.

All of these items can be purchased inexpensively at your local supermarket or department store. With a food scale, however, you'd be wise to spend more money and purchase a battery-operated digital scale instead of the less expensive, spring-loaded type.

Take a Vitamin-Mineral Tablet Each Day

When on a reduced-calorie eating plan, it's a good idea to take one multiple vitamin with minerals tablet each morning with breakfast. Make sure no nutri-

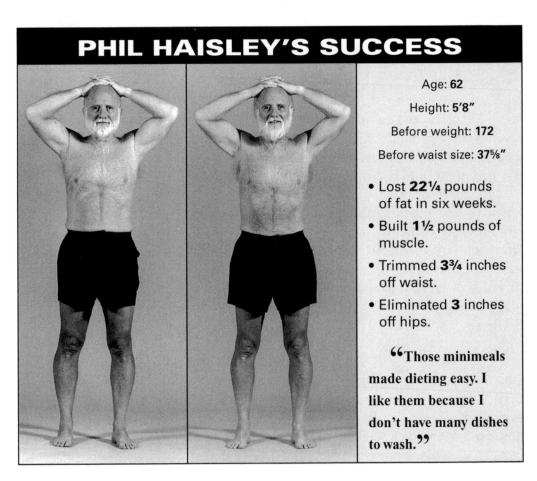

PHIL HAISLEY'S SUCCESS

Age: **62**

Height: **5'8"**

Before weight: **172**

Before waist size: **37⅝"**

- Lost **22¼ pounds** of fat in six weeks.
- Built **1½ pounds of** muscle.
- Trimmed **3¾ inches** off waist.
- Eliminated **3 inches** off hips.

"Those minimeals made dieting easy. I like them because I don't have many dishes to wash."

ent listed on the label exceeds 100 percent of the Recommended Dietary Allowances. High-potency supplements are not necessary.

Examine Menus and Shopping List

Look through the ASAP menus and shopping list in chapter 10 for a preview of what you'll be eating during the six-week course. Your results will be more effective if you plan ahead.

Prepare for Superhydration

The drinking of at least one gallon of ice-cold water each day is an integral component of the ASAP course. For the first two weeks, men start with 128 ounces per day, while women begin with 160 ounces per day. After the first two weeks, both women and men raise their water drinking by 16 ounces per week. Here's the way the week-by-week guidelines progress:

WEEK-BY-WEEK GUIDELINES					
Weeks	1 & 2	3	4	5	6
Superhydrating (ounces per day)					
Women	160	176	192	208	224
Men	128	144	160	176	192

Why do I recommend 32 ounces more water per day for a woman than a man? My studies reveal that most women suffer from fluid retention at various times of the month. Such fluid retention tends to negate weight loss. An extra quart of water speeds circulation and helps the typical woman prevent fluid accumulation.

Women progress up to 224 ounces, or 1¾ gallons, of water per day during the sixth week. Men drink slightly less: 192 ounces, or 1½ gallons, per day during the last week of the course.

The secret to drinking this much water each day is to sip it continually rather than pour it down in sizable gulps. A 32-ounce, insulated plastic bottle with a straw—which is an inexpensive purchase at most discount department stores—makes it easier to comply with the recommendations. Thus, you'll be able to carry your bottle with you throughout the day and sip from it frequently.

Another helpful superhydration tip is to consume 75 to 80 percent of your quota before 5:00 P.M. Participants in my ASAP course find that it's easier to drink early in the day than it is to drink late at night. To keep track of your water drinking, place rubber bands around the bottom of the bottle equal to the number of bottles or quarts you are supposed to sip. Each time you complete 32 ounces, take off a rubber band and put it in your pocket.

For the first two weeks or so, your bladder will be hypersensitive to the increased amount of fluid. Most people find that they have to urinate from fifteen to twenty times a day during the initial weeks. Soon your bladder will adapt and you will urinate less frequently but in larger volumes.

Superhydration may be inconvenient for a while. But the inconvenience is justified if you realize that you are expediting the fat-loss process each time you transfer heat calories out of your body.

Get Better Quality Sleep Each Night

I hope by now you've thought about the guidelines presented in chapter 7 for improving your sleeping habits. If you need extra sleep, then do whatever is necessary to retire ninety minutes earlier each night. Getting higher-quality rest will accentuate your fat-loss and muscle-building results.

Consider Other Synergistic Activities

The *big three* in synergy are eating, strength training, and superhydrating. In chapter 8, I discussed other activities that heighten your results from the ASAP program. It will be to your advantage to include as many of these activities— such as walking after your evening meal, practicing a stomach vacuum, and staying uncomfortably cool—as you can over the six-week course. Don't neglect the little things, like using color wisely, cutting back on evening TV, and emphasizing good posture. They can all add up and make a big difference in the degree of your success.

Be Excited, but Be Patient

You are now well prepared to begin *A Flat Stomach ASAP.* You should be ready. You should be excited.

But you also must be patient. Permanent change takes time. The ASAP course will make a difference in your life.

Let's get started.

10

ACTION:

PRACTICE THIS EATING PLAN

In 1985, I had great success with my Nautilus diet program by providing participants with a lot of general guidelines centered around food substitutions. The participants were supplied with two charts that described how they could mix servings using the basic food groups to equal the required number of daily calories.

Along with these flexible guidelines were dozens of recipes. In fact, the complete diet contained seventy-two recipes, some of which took more than one hour to fix. People liked to cook and spend time in the kitchen in those days.

When Nautilus Sports/Medical Industries relocated its headquarters to Dallas, Texas, in 1987, I took the Nautilus diet with me. Within weeks after I introduced the program to the metro-Dallas area, I began to see frustrated dieters. Some complained about all the choices. Others griped about the cooking involved. Yet others wanted microwavable foods and prepackaged meals. There seemed to be general agreement that, while the diet certainly worked, it was too complex and too time-consuming.

The men and women in Dallas wanted simplicity, convenience, and speed. Being of similar mind-set, I valued what these people were saying.

As a result, I went back to the drawing board. I consulted several dieticians. I spent more time in the supermarket examining the latest frozen foods. I experimented more with microwave cooking. I studied the current food science journals.

I soon had a new batch of menus and recipes. And I made the substitutions more specific.

Almost every six weeks, I'd test more new menus and recipes on another group of dieters in Dallas. Gradually, winning combinations began to emerge.

I moved back to Florida in 1991. At the Gainesville Health & Fitness Center, where I did the original research for the Nautilus diet, I applied the revised eating plan. With a few adaptations, I was soon recording almost the same fat-loss results in six weeks that I had previously achieved in ten weeks.

Every year since then, the fat-loss results—because of the continuous feedback, adjustments, and retesting—have gotten better and better. The culmination of all this research is included in *A Flat Stomach ASAP*.

Simple, Convenient, and Fast

Everyone likes to see fast results when they start a diet and exercise course. When I worked with Don Brown on the AB Trainer infomercial, which I referred to in chapter 1, we developed the "10-Day Quick-Start Program for a Flat Stomach." During the research phase, I supervised subjects through this ten-day plan with dramatic results. The men lost an average of eleven pounds of fat and the women lost an average of seven pounds. Both the men and women dropped an average of 2½ inches off their waist.

It seemed obvious that I should revise and expand the ten-day plan and make it the first two weeks of a more comprehensive six-week program. That's exactly what I did, while keeping the Quick-Start headline still prominent.

Women begin the Quick Start with five minimeals that total 1,100 calories a day. Men start with 1,300 calories a day.

After the Quick Start, the calories increase by 200 for week 3, and then descend by 100 calories each week until the end of week 6.

WEEK-BY-WEEK-GUIDELINES					
Weeks	1 & 2	3	4	5	6
Eating (calories per day)					
Women	1,100	1,300	1,200	1,100	1,000
Men	1,300	1,500	1,400	1,300	1,200

Important: Men over six feet two inches tall and weighing more than 250 pounds need 300 calories added to their daily totals; very active men require 300 more calories per day; and vegetarians apply a list of meat substitutions. Please refer to chapter 12 for complete details.

I've tried to keep current on the popular brand names and calorie counts, which are listed in the following menus. But as you probably know, products are sometimes changed or discontinued. If a listed brand is not available in your area, you'll have to substitute a similar product. Become a keen reader of labels. Ask questions about any food or notation you don't understand. Supermarket managers usually are helpful. If they don't have the answers to your questions, they will research them for you.

Each day you'll choose a limited selection of foods for breakfast and lunch. I've found that most dieters can consume the same basic breakfast and basic

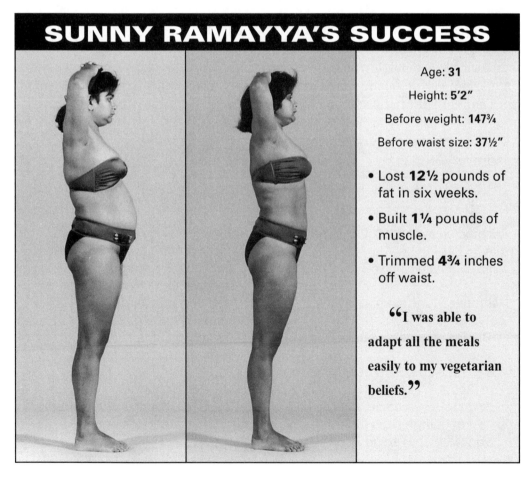

SUNNY RAMAYYA'S SUCCESS

Age: **31**

Height: **5'2"**

Before weight: **147¾**

Before waist size: **37½"**

- Lost **12½** pounds of fat in six weeks.

- Built **1¼** pounds of muscle.

- Trimmed **4¾** inches off waist.

"I was able to adapt all the meals easily to my vegetarian beliefs."

lunch for months with no modification. A little variety during the evening meal, however, will make daily eating interesting and enjoyable. Also, the eating plan includes an afternoon and an evening minimeal to keep your hunger at a low level.

You'll always have a 300-calorie breakfast, lunch, and dinner. Only your snack calories will change: men—from 400 to 600 to 500 to 400 to 300 calories per day; women—from 200 to 400 to 300 to 200 to 100 calories per day.

Most important, you'll find that everything has been simplified so even the most kitchen-inept person can succeed. Very little cooking is required. All you have to do is read the following menus, examine the shopping list, select and purchase your food choices, and follow the directions. It's just that simple.

The Quick-Start menus are classified as no-frills. Their simplicity is one reason why they work so well. A few more choices will be added for weeks three, four, five, and six. But you'll still be applying the basic Quick-Start menus. Many of my ASAP participants, in fact, have used the basic menus for six months or longer.

Let's have a look at the menus, beginning with the two-week Quick Start. Calories for each food are noted in parentheses. Then study carefully the Guidelines and Substitutions.

ASAP QUICK-START MENUS
WEEKS 1 & 2

Women consume 1,100 calories per day.
Men consume 1,300 calories per day.

Minimeal 1. Breakfast = 300 calories
Choice of bagel or shake.
Bagel:
1 plain bagel, Sara Lee, frozen (210)
½ ounce light cream cheese (30)
½ cup orange juice (55)
noncaloric beverage

Shake:
2 packets of Perfect Score shake mix (300), or other meal replacements to equal the appropriate calories
14 ounces cold water
Place ingredients in shaker or blender, mix until smooth.

Minimeal 2. Lunch = 300 calories
Choice of sandwich or shake.
Sandwich:
2 slices whole-wheat bread (140)

1 tablespoon Smart Beat Super
Light Margarine (20)
1 teaspoon Dijon mustard (0)
(optional)
2 ounces white meat (about 8 thin
slices) chicken or turkey (80)
1 ounce fat-free cheese (1½ slices)
(50)
noncaloric beverage

Shake:
2 packets of Perfect Score shake
mix (300), or other meal
replacements to equal the
appropriate calories
14 ounces cold water
Place ingredients in shaker or
blender, mix until smooth.

Minimeal 3. Afternoon snack = 100/200 calories

Women have one selection; men
have both.
   1 apple (3-inch diameter) (100)
   1 cup light, nonfat, flavored yogurt
   (100)

Minimeal 4. Dinner = 300 calories

Choice of one of three frozen,
microwavable meals:
- Lasagna with Vegetables,
Michelina's (260)
½ cup skim milk (45)
Noncaloric beverage
- Traditional Beef Tips, Healthy
Choice (260)
½ cup skim milk (45)
Noncaloric beverage

- Glazed Chicken (Chicken
Tenderloins with Vegetable
Rice), Lean Cuisine (240)
⅔ cup skim milk (60)
Noncaloric beverage

Minimeal 5. Evening snack = 100/200 calories

Women have one selection, men
have both.
   1 apple (3-inch diameter) (100)
   1 cup light, nonfat, flavored yogurt
   (100)

Notes

Noncaloric beverages are any type
of water—tap, bottled, carbonated,
or flavored—with no calories. Other
noncaloric beverages are soft drinks
with zero calories and no caffeine,
and decaffeinated teas and coffees.

Perfect Score is the only meal
replacement on the market that
meets my ideal macronutrient
composition of 60 percent
carbohydrates, 20 percent fats, and
20 percent proteins. You may
purchase Perfect Score by calling
(888) 256-2727.

ASAP GUIDELINES AND SUBSTITUTIONS FOR WEEKS 3, 4, 5, AND 6

Women

Week 3 = 1,300 calories a day:
Add two snacks (+ 200 calories) to
basic Quick-Start menus.

Week 4 = 1,200 calories a day:
Eliminate one snack (− 100
calories) from week 3.

Week 5 = 1,100 calories a day:
Eliminate one snack (− 100
calories) from week 4.

Week 6 = 1,000 calories a day:
Eliminate one snack (− 100
calories) from week 5.

Men

Week 3 = 1,500 calories a day:
Add three slices whole-wheat
bread (+ 210 calories) to basic
Quick-Start menus.

Week 4 = 1,400 calories a day:
Eliminate one snack (− 100
calories) from week 3.

Week 5 = 1,300 calories a day:
Eliminate one snack (− 100
calories) from week 4.

Week 6 = 1,200 calories a day:
Eliminate one snack (− 100
calories) from week 5.

**One of the following may be
substituted for a 300-calorie lunch:**
Soup:
Healthy Choice Chicken Pasta, 15-
ounce can (240)
1 slice whole-wheat bread (70)
noncaloric beverage

Chef salad:
In a large bowl, mix the following:
2 cups lettuce, chopped (20)
2 ounces white meat chicken or
turkey (80)
2 ounces fat-free cheese (100)
4 slices tomato, chopped (28)
1 tablespoon fat-free dressing (6)
1 slice whole-wheat bread (70)
noncaloric beverage

**One of the following may be
substituted for a 100-calorie snack:**
- 5 dried prunes (100)
- 1 ounce raisins (82)
- ½ cantaloupe (5-inch diameter)
(94)
- 1 large banana (100)
- 2 cups light, microwave popcorn
(100)

**One of the following may be
substituted for a 300-calorie
dinner:**
- Beef Stroganoff, Budget
Gourmet (290)
noncaloric beverage

- Lean 'n Tasty Macaroni & Cheese, Michelina's (290)
  noncaloric beverage
- Country Inn Roast Turkey, Healthy Choice (250)
  ½ cup skim milk (45)
  noncaloric beverage
- Tuna salad
  In a large bowl, mix the following:

1 6-ounce can chunk light tuna in water (180)
¼ cup (2 ounces) whole kernel corn, canned, no salt added (30)
2 tablespoons sweet pickle relish (40)
1 tablespoon Hellmann's Light Mayonnaise (50)
1 tablespoon Dijon mustard (0)

Shopping List

The quantities you'll need for the listed foods will depend on your specific selections. Review your choices and adjust the shopping list accordingly. Remember to check nutrition information on products you buy so that you can carefully follow the serving sizes in the menus. It may be helpful for you to photocopy this list each week before doing your shopping.

Staples
orange juice
skim milk
meal replacement shakes
whole-wheat bread
Smart Beat Super Light Margarine
fat-free salad dressing
Hellmann's Light Mayonnaise
Dijon mustard
noncaloric beverages: water, diet soft drinks, decaffeinated tea and coffee

Grains
Sara Lee bagels, frozen
popcorn, microwave light

Fruits
bananas, small and large
apples (3-inch diameter)
cantaloupes (5-inch diameter)
dried prunes
raisins

Vegetables
>lettuce
>tomatoes
>whole-kernel corn, canned, no salt added
>sweet pickle relish

Dairy
>yogurt, nonfat light
>cream cheese, light
>cheese, fat-free

Meat, Poultry, Fish, and Entrées
>chicken, thin sliced
>turkey, thin sliced
>tuna, canned chunk light in water
>canned soup: Healthy Choice Chicken Pasta
>frozen microwavable dinners or entrées
>- Michelina's Lasagna with Vegetables
>- Healthy Choice Traditional Beef Tips
>- Lean Cuisine Glazed Chicken
>- Budget Gourmet Beef Stroganoff
>- Michelina's Lean 'n Tasty Macaroni & Cheese
>- Healthy Choice Country Inn Roast Turkey

11

ACCELERATION:

Use This Strength-Training Routine

know you're anxious to begin the recommended strength-training routine. And you won't be disappointed. This routine will most definitely accelerate your mobilization of fat. But before you start, there are still a few salient points that you need to review and understand.

Spot Reduction of Fat: Not Possible

Many people believe that when you exercise a specific body part, such as the stomach or abdominals, the involved muscles burn the surrounding fat for energy. This belief is the primary reason high-repetition sit-ups and leg raises are practiced as a method to remove fat from the waist.

If spot reduction of fat was possible, then people who chew gum regularly would have skinny faces. But such is not the case.

No direct pathways exist from the muscle cells to the fat cells. When fat is used for energy, it is mobilized primarily through the liver from multiple fat cells all over the body.

Possible: Spot Production of Strength

While spot reduction of fat from your waist is not going to happen, spot production of strength, tightness, and firmness is possible and highly recommended. One of your goals is to make your midsection muscles—rectus abdominis, external oblique, internal oblique, and transverse abdominis—significantly stronger, which in turn will make your entire waistline area tighter and firmer.

Muscle Isolation

The strength-training routine illustrated in this chapter isolates and intensely works your abdominals, but it does not neglect other major muscles. You'll also be working your hips, thighs, shoulders, back, chest, and arms.

If you combine this strength-training routine with the diet plan, the super-hydration schedule, and the other steps in this course, then you've done everything practical—just short of surgery—to maximize stomach flattening.

Precision Basics

Read through first. Spend several minutes examining the exercises in this chapter. Read the instructions carefully. Practice will perfect your movements, but for now, do them as best you can.

No special equipment. The strength-training routine in this chapter is designed to be used with no special equipment, in the privacy of your home. If you already have a roller-type abdominal machine, then I'll show you how to incorporate it into your routine. Or if you are a member of a commercial fitness center, a YMCA, or any facility that has heavy-duty strength-training equipment, I'll give you the specifics on how to use these machines—see chapter 12—in the most efficient way. You'll soon find that the equipment is not nearly as important as the way in which you use it. Remember, controlled movement is the mandate.

Apply super-slow repetitions. Rushing through each strength-training exercise diminishes effects and can result in injury. Each repetition, with one or two exceptions, should take approximately ten seconds on the lifting and five seconds on the lowering. If in doubt about your speed of movement, always move slower rather than faster.

Emphasize breathing. Try not to hold your breath on any repetition. Keep your mouth open and breathe. When the movement gets difficult, purse your lips and exhale in short bursts—just like they teach in a Lamaze class.

Count the repetitions. Start with four repetitions on most exercises, then at each successive workout, increase the repetitions by one. Thus if you start your workout on a Monday, the progression would be as follows:

Week 1
Monday—4 repetitions
Wednesday—5 repetitions
Friday—6 repetitions

Week 2
Monday—7 repetitions
Wednesday—8 repetitions
Friday—Add resistance and make harder.

After you can do eight or more perfect repetitions, you must add approximately 5 percent more resistance to your body. This in turn will reduce your repetitions down to four or five at the next workout. Then, it's your job to progress up to eight repetitions once again, and add another 5 percent, and so on.

Focus your concentration. Proper strength training is both physical and mental. If you direct your attention to the muscles you're targeting, then your results will improve. If it's a trunk curl, for example, focus on the front abdominals. Try to visualize them shortening each time you lift your shoulders. If it's a side bend, focus on mobilizing your oblique muscles to their maximum. Aim your mind like a laser beam. The effect will amaze you.

Anticipate some soreness. Soreness in your body is an indicator that you've contracted and stretched some underutilized muscles. Expect some tenderness after your first workout, especially on the front and sides of your waist. Don't fret. Your second workout will ease the soreness, and it should be gone by your third strength-training session.

Warm up and cool down. Before strength training, take several minutes to warm up. A good way to do this is to walk in place. Start lifting your feet and hands in a slow, walking-in-place motion. After one minute, gradually increase the range by lifting your hands to the level of your ears. Practice this exaggerated action for another minute. After your workout, cool down by walking around the exercise area, getting a drink of water, and moving your arms in slow circles. Continue these easy actions for several minutes until your heart rate slows down.

At-Home, Strength-Training Routine

The Quick Start is your first schedule and it involves only five strength-training exercises. Thereafter through week 6, you will add one exercise per week to your basic five. Here's a listing of each schedule.

AT-HOME, ASAP STRENGTH-TRAINING ROUTINE		
Quick Start Weeks 1 & 2	**Week 3**	**Week 4**
1. Trunk Curl	1. Trunk Curl	1. Trunk Curl
2. Trunk Curl with Twist	2. Trunk Curl with Twist	2. Trunk Curl with Twist
3. Side Bend	3. Side Bend	3. Side Bend
4. Wall Squat	4. Wall Squat	4. Wall Squat
5. Negative Push-Up	5. Negative Push-Up	5. Negative Push-Up
	6. Reverse Trunk Curl*	6. Reverse Trunk Curl
		7. Lateral Raise with Weight*
Week 5	**Week 6**	
1. Trunk Curl	1. Trunk Curl	
2. Trunk Curl with Twist	2. Trunk Curl with Twist	
3. Side Bend	3. Side Bend	
4. Wall Squat	4. Wall Squat	
5. Negative Push-Up	5. Negative Push-Up	
6. Reverse Trunk Curl	6. Reverse Trunk Curl	
7. Lateral Raise with Weight	7. Lateral Raise with Weight	
8. Pullover with Weight*	8. Pullover with Weight	
	9. Biceps Curl with Weight*	

*New exercise

A description of each at-home, strength-training exercise follows:

HAND POSITIONS ON THE TRUNK CURL

Where you place your hands and arms during the trunk curl and the trunk curl with twist can make the exercise easier or harder.

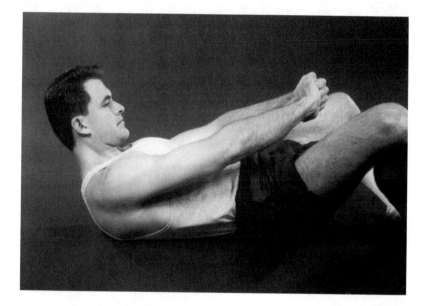

The basic, learning position is with your arms extended over your navel and your hands clasped. This places some of the weight of your hands and arms forward, which decreases the resistance of your torso. Everyone should master the trunk curl initially from this position.

(continued)

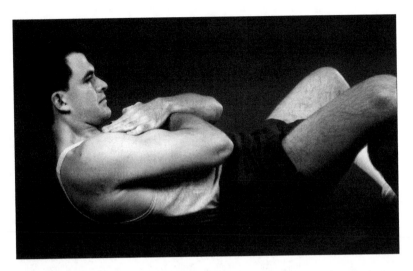

The first progression for a harder trunk curl is to cross your hands over your chest. This moves some of the weight of your hands and arms from your navel to your chest, thus adding more resistance to your torso.

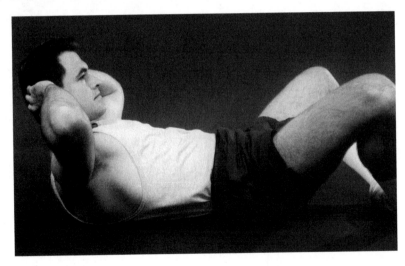

The second progression is to shift the weight of your hands and arms from your chest to your head area. Do not interlace your hands behind your head or neck. Doing so with your hands can possibly strain your neck by pulling forward on your head. Instead, cup your hands around your ears while keeping your elbows back and at shoulder level. Your hands and arms in this position make the trunk curl significantly harder than the first two versions.

The third progression (not pictured) requires that you hold with your hands a weight plate flat across your chest. As this style gets easier, you simply increase the poundage of the weight plate.

Trunk Curl
(for midsection)

Starting position. Lie faceup on the floor. Bring your heels up close to your buttocks. Put the soles of your feet together and spread your knees wide. Where you place your hands and arms can make the movement easier or harder. The positions (in the order of difficulty) are arms extended and fingers interlaced in front of your navel, arms crossed over your chest, arms spread above shoulders with hands cupping your ears. Begin with your arms extended and fingers interlaced in front of your navel.

Movement. Focus on curling your head, shoulders, and upper back off the floor—ever so slowly. Reach with your hands through your thighs, at the same time curling your shoulders upward. Try to achieve your highest upper-back-off-the-floor position at the count of ten. Pause briefly in the top position. Lower your back and shoulders smoothly to the floor in five seconds. Feel your upper back, shoulders, and head come in contact with the floor, but do not relax or rest. Touch, then barely move again in the upward direction. Continue for the required repetitions. When you can do eight repetitions of the trunk curl in perfect form, progress to the next hardest positioning of your arms. Cross your arms over your chest, reduce your repetitions, and work upward from four once again.

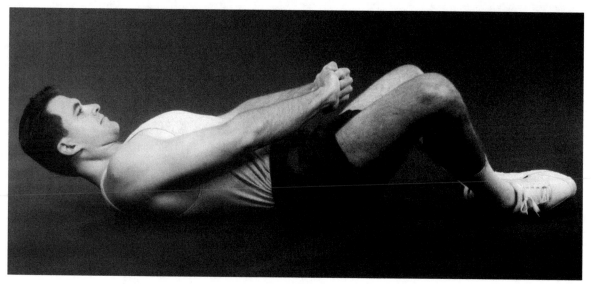

Trunk curl, starting position: Initiate movement by lifting your head off the floor. Then, curl your shoulders and reach with your hands toward your feet.

Trunk Curl with Twist
(for middle and sides)

Starting position. Lie faceup on the floor and assume the same position as you did for the trunk curl.

Movement. Curl your head, shoulders, and upper back off the floor slowly. Instead of reaching with your hands through your open thighs, twist smoothly to the left and try to touch your left knee with your hands. Remember, this is a deliberate ten-second movement. Pause in this top position. Lower your right shoulder to the floor in five seconds. But do not relax. Repeat the twisting to your left knee for the required repetitions. Rest for a few seconds, then perform the movement to your right knee in a similar manner.

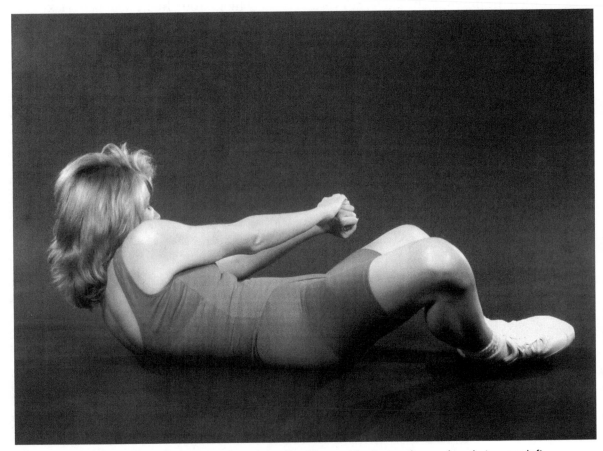

Trunk curl with twist to left: Raise your right shoulder and try to touch your hands to your left knee.

On the next training day, work your right side before your left side. Continue to alternate between starting on your left side, or starting on your right side. Avoid beginning on the same side for two consecutive workouts.

When you can perform eight repetitions of the trunk curl with twist to both sides, progress to the next hardest position of your arms, and work upward from four repetitions.

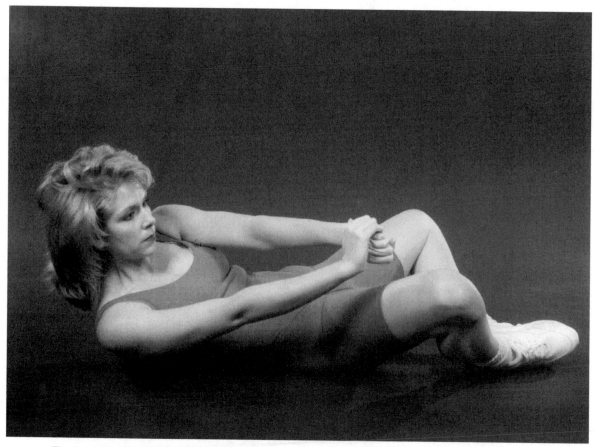

Trunk curl with twist to right: Focus on slowly contracting your midsection muscles as you reach toward your right knee.

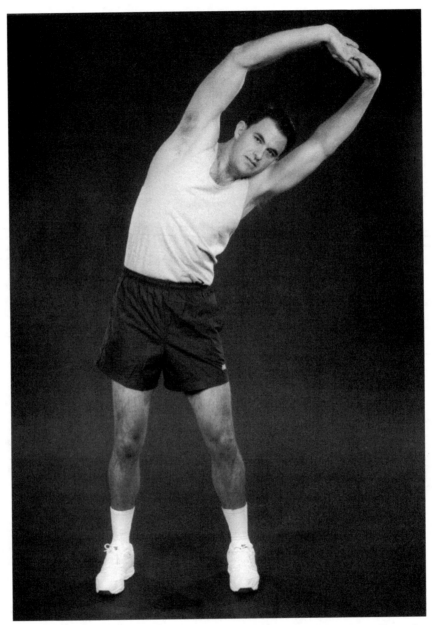

Side bend to left: Reach toward the ceiling first and then bend laterally to the left. You'll feel this movement in your right side muscles.

Side Bend
(for sides of waist)

Starting position. Stand with your feet hip-width apart. Extend your arms above your head and interlace your fingers.

Movement. Stand tall and reach toward the ceiling. When you achieve the maximum height, start bending laterally to the left. Pause briefly in the stretched position and reach again with your arms and hands, this time maximally to the left. This bending and reaching should take five seconds. Return slowly to the top center position in ten seconds. Do not let your hands move forward. Keep them extended and directly over the middle of your head. Reach toward the ceiling with both hands and repeat bending to the left side for the required repetitions. Rest for a few seconds with your arms hanging at your sides. Then perform the movement to your right side in a similar manner for the same number of repetitions.

During your next training session, remember to work your right side before your left side. Continue this alternating process. When you can perform eight repetitions of the side bend to both sides, add a 2½-pound weight to your hands and work upward from four repetitions.

The super-slow protocol, when applied to the next two exercises—the wall squat and the push-up—makes their difficulty more than most people can master. Thus the wall squat and the negative push-up are performed in a slightly different style than super slow. The wall squat uses a sustained contraction, where you'll be holding a midrange position for ten seconds. The negative push-up emphasizes a ten-second lowering and an assisted way of getting back to the top.

Wall Squat
(for buttocks and thighs)

Starting position. Stand erect and lean back against a smooth, sturdy wall. Place your heels three inches wider apart than your hips and approximately twelve inches away from where the wall touches the floor. Rest your hands on your hips.

Movement. Slide your back down the wall until the tops of your thighs are parallel to the floor. Hold this parallel level for ten seconds. Push back to the top position but avoid locking your knees. Keep them slightly bent. Immediately lower to the parallel position and hold for another ten seconds. Push back and repeat for six sustained-contraction repetitions.

With the wall squat, your goal is to do six thirty-second-hold repetitions. In other words, you keep your repetitions constant at six, and gradually extend your time of contraction. Increase the duration of each repetition by one second each workout for the first several weeks. Then try to add two seconds to each repetition. Before the end of six weeks, you should be able to achieve six thirty-second repetitions. When that time occurs, you need to do the movement with a couple of small weights in your hands.

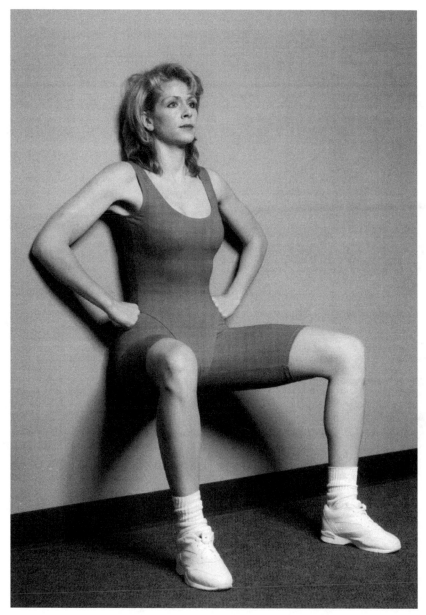

Wall squat, bottom position: Make sure the tops of your thighs are parallel to the floor and your shins are parallel to the wall. This results in a ninety-degree bend in your hips and your knees.

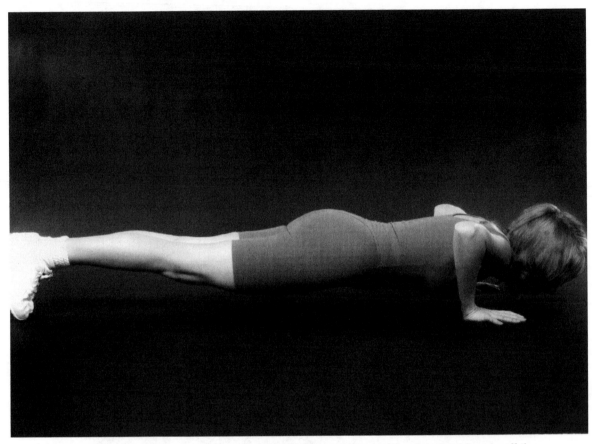

Negative push-up, bottom position: Hold the down position—with your chest barely off the floor—for several seconds, if you can. This is the most productive part of the movement, so emphasize it.

Negative Push-Up
(for chest, shoulders, and backs of upper arms)

Starting position. Assume a standard push-up position on your toes and hands with your arms straight and your body stiff. If it is too difficult for you to hold this position, then you can balance on your knees rather than on your toes.

Movement. Lower your body to the floor by bending your arms. You should be halfway down in five seconds and almost all the way down in eight or nine seconds. Touch the floor with your chest at the ten-second mark. Do *not* push yourself up to the top position. Use your legs to get up. Place your knees on the floor, raise your chest, straighten your arms, and slide back on your toes. Presto! You're in the top position. Repeat for four negative-only, or lowering, repetitions. Add one repetition per workout.

When you can do eight negative-only push-ups in perfect form, try doing the positive movement. Push your body up by straightening your arms. In other words, you'll now be performing the pushing up as well as the lowering. Gradually progress into the super-slow style: ten seconds up and five seconds down. Eight super-slow push-ups is your goal.

Reverse Trunk Curl
(for lower abdominals)

Starting position. Lie faceup on the floor with your hands, palms down, on either side of your hips. Bring your thighs to your chest so your hips and thighs are in a flexed position. During the movement, it's important to try to keep your thighs near your chest.

Movement. This contraction is the opposite of the trunk curl. Instead of curling your shoulders, you'll be raising your hips. Curl your hips toward your

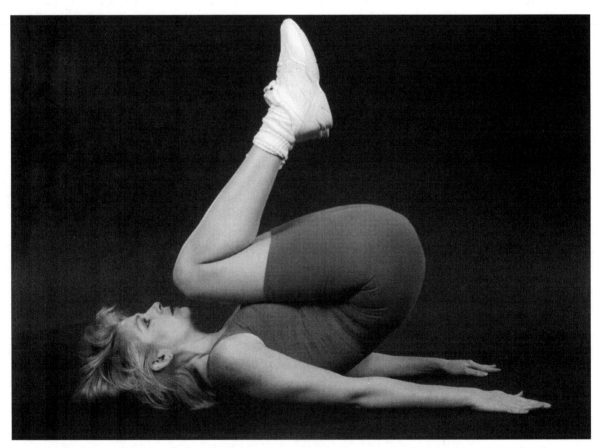

Reverse trunk curl, top position: Notice that the angle between the floor and your lower back is approximately forty-five degrees. Keep your thighs near your chest as you lower your hips back to the starting position.

chest by gradually lifting your buttocks and lower back off the floor. To counter-balance your hips, push down on the floor with your hands. Once you get the hang of this movement, your hips and lower back should be at a forty-five-degree angle to the floor in the top position. Practice moving to the top position slowly in ten seconds. Lower your hips smoothly to the floor in five seconds. Try not to cheat by moving your feet or knees. Repeat for the required repetitions.

This is probably the most difficult abdominal exercise to master in this routine. Once you perform eight super-slow repetitions in perfect form, you can make the movement harder by adding ankle weights to your feet.

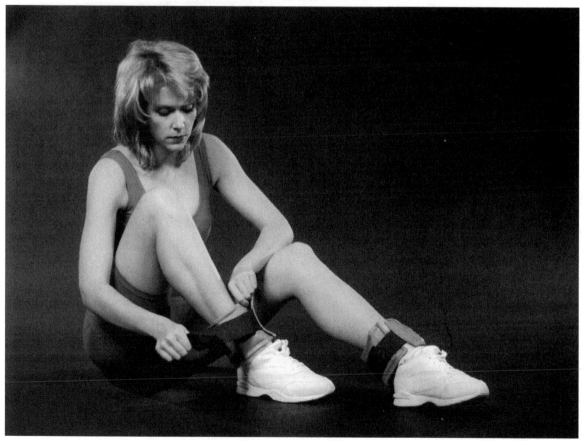

When you can perform eight repetitions of the reverse trunk curl in perfect form, ankle weights will make the exercise more challenging.

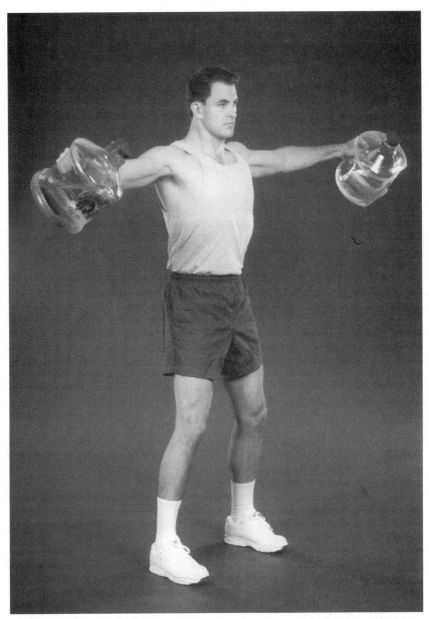

Lateral raise with water bottles, top position: Large water bottles, milk jugs, or dumbbells work well for this exercise. Pause when your arms are parallel to the floor or slightly above. Ease out of the top position smoothly and under control.

Lateral Raise with Weight
(for shoulders)

Starting position. Grasp a light dumbbell in each hand and stand. If you don't have access to adjustable dumbbells, use two plastic bottles with sculptured handles. The one-gallon size full of water weighs about eight pounds. The weight can be lowered by using less water. Lock your elbows and wrists and keep them locked throughout the movement. All the action should occur around your shoulder joints.

Movement. Raise your arms sideways. Try to reach the top position, where the dumbbells are level with your ears, in ten seconds. Make sure your elbows remain locked. Pause. Lower your arms smoothly to your sides in five seconds. Do not rest. Continue the movement for the required repetitions. If you can do eight or more repetitions, increase the resistance by 5 percent at your next workout.

Pullover with Weight
(for upper back and chest)

Starting position. Lie crossways on a bench with your shoulders in contact with the bench and your head and lower body off the bench. Hold a dumbbell on one end in both hands and position it over your chest with your arms straight. If you don't have a dumbbell, use two plastic bottles containing water and hold one in each hand.

Movement. Take a deep breath and lower the dumbbell smoothly behind your head in five seconds. Keep your elbows straight and stretch briefly. Lift the dumbbell slowly back to the starting position in ten seconds. Repeat for the required repetitions. Add 5 percent more resistance when you can perform eight repetitions in correct form.

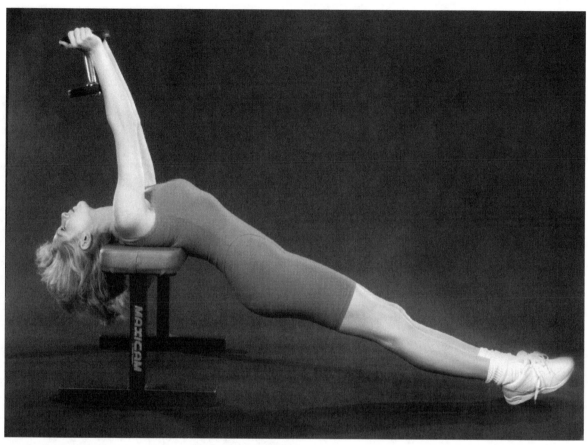

Pullover with dumbbell, top position: Expand your chest and lower the dumbbell smoothly behind your head for a full stretch. Keep your elbows straight as you move your arms.

Biceps Curl with Weight
(for front upper arms)

Starting position. Grasp a dumbbell in each hand and stand. If you don't have access to dumbbells, use two plastic bottles filled with the appropriate amount of water. Anchor your elbows firmly against the sides of your waist and keep them there throughout the movement. Lean slightly forward with your shoulders.

Movement. Look down at your hands and curl the weight slowly in ten seconds. Pause in the top position, but do not move your elbows forward. Keep your hands in front of your elbows. Lower the dumbbells smoothly in five seconds. Again, keep your elbows stable against your sides. Repeat for the required number of repetitions. When you can do eight super-slow repetitions in proper form, add 5 percent more resistance.

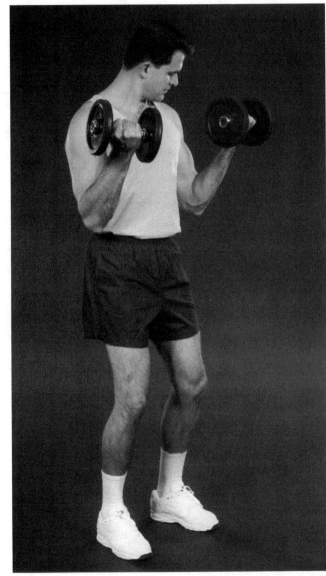

Biceps curl with dumbbells, top position: Anchor your elbows by your sides as you arc the dumbbells smoothly to the bottom.

Home Abdominal Machines

As I mentioned in the introduction, more than six million people in the United States have purchased home abdominal machines. Perhaps you were one of these people. If so, great! I want you to get it handy. You'll probably be able to use it according to the prescribed super-slow style.

I'm most familiar with the AB Trainer, which supplies roller-frame support for your head, neck, shoulders, and arms. If you'd like to order an AB Trainer, please call 800-619-4227.

Most of the other home abdominal machines, and there are more than a dozen of them, are designed around the same basic principles. First, the frame that surrounds your upper body supports and stabilizes your head and neck, as well as your shoulders and arms. This allows you to isolate your abdominals better by eliminating much of your upper body from the exercise movements. Second, the rolling frame varies the resistance that is placed on your contracting abdominal muscles. In other words, the overload on your muscles is more effective. The resistance is heavier in your stronger positions and lighter in your weaker positions.

So if you have one of the home abdominal machines that is designed around the roller frame, by all means use it. But use it according to the super-slow style.

Look back at the listing of the strength-training routine on page 102. The exercise that I want you to do with your home abdominal machine will replace the following: trunk curl, trunk curl with twist, and reverse trunk curl. Instead of these exercises, you will do the *basic crunch* and the *side crunch* in the one and two slots, and the *reverse crunch* in the six position.

Here's the way to apply super slow to these abdominal machine exercises:

Basic Crunch with Home Abdominal Machine
(for midsection)

Starting position. Place the home abdominal machine on a flat, stable floor. A mat or rug may be situated under the machine for comfort. Sit in front of the rocker system and scoot backward into the machine. Ease the back of your head onto the head pad. Bend your knees and bring your knees close to your buttocks. Your shoulders should be on the floor. Reach up with both arms and place them behind the curved bar. Stabilize your arms and shoulders.

Movement. Contract your abdominals gradually by shortening the distance between your breastbone and navel. At the same time, push forward slowly with your hands on the top of the machine. Crunch your abdominals into their fully shortened position. This entire process should take ten seconds. Do not move your chin toward your chest. Keep your neck and face relaxed. Pause briefly in the top position. Lower your shoulders smoothly to the floor in five seconds. Do not rest. Barely crunch ever so slowly. Repeat for the required repetitions.

You can make working out on your home abdominal machine progressively more challenging by adding small weight plates to the bars on either side of the head pad. Or you can make your own weights by placing heavy objects or materials (such as sand) in old socks and tying them onto the bottom bars.

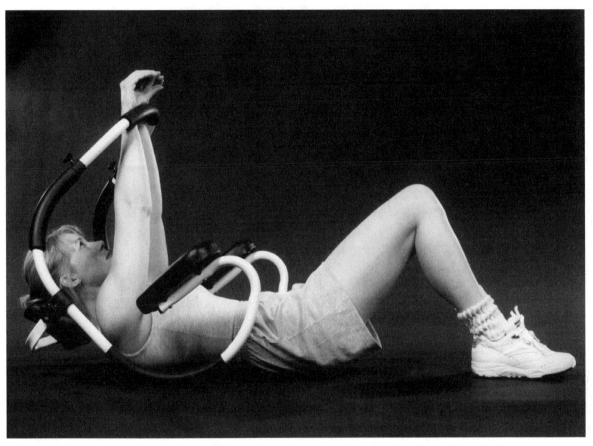

Basic crunch with AB Trainer, starting position: Push the curved bar forward by slowly contracting your abdominals. Keep your neck relaxed during the movement.

Side Crunch with Home Abdominal Machine
(for middle and sides of waist)

Starting position. Assume the same posture as for the basic crunch, except rotate your hips to the right. Your left knee should now be on top of your right knee. Keep your shoulders on the floor. Cross your left hand over your right hand.

Movement. Push forward slowly with your hands and curl your shoulders off the floor as far as possible in ten seconds. You'll feel an intense contraction in the left side of your waist. Pause briefly in the top position. Lower your shoulders smoothly to the floor in five seconds. Repeat for the required repetitions. Rest for a few seconds, rotate your hips to the left, then perform the side crunch for your right side.

On the next training day, work your right side before your left side. Continue to alternate between starting on your left side, or starting on your right side. Avoid beginning on the same side for two consecutive workouts. When you can do eight repetitions of the side crunch in both directions, add a small amount of weight to the back of the machine and work upward from four repetitions.

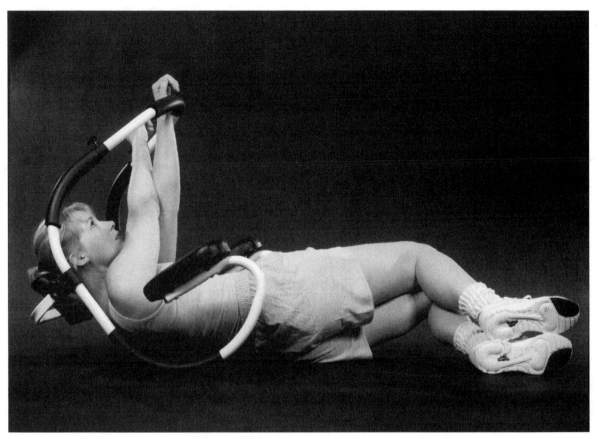

Side crunch to right with AB Trainer, midrange position: Roll slowly into a full contraction of your right side abdominals.

Reverse Crunch with Home Abdominal Machine
(for lower abdomen)

Starting position. Assume the same posture as for the basic crunch, except flex your hips and bring your thighs and knees near your chest. With your hips flexed, push forward with your hands and slightly lift your shoulders off the floor. This is your starting position.

Movement. Without moving your shoulders or knees, curl your buttocks off the floor slowly in ten seconds. You'll only be able to lift your hips through a short range, but if you do it correctly, you'll really feel it under your navel. Pause briefly at the top. Lower your buttocks smoothly to the starting position in five seconds. Focus intensely on lifting and lowering only your hips and bringing your lower abdomen into action. Repeat for the required repetitions. Once you work up to eight super-slow repetitions in the reverse crunch, you can make the movement harder by adding ankle weights to your feet.

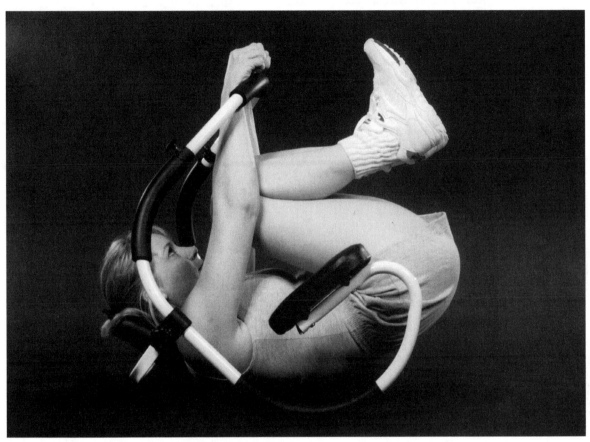

Reverse crunch with AB Trainer, top position: Hold this contraction briefly and you'll feel it intensely in the muscles underneath your navel.

Accurate Record Keeping

It is essential that you keep accurate records of all your strength-training sessions. Make three photocopies of the chart that follows. Each photocopy contains enough space to record your workouts for two weeks. List your exercises for each segment in the left column. Record each workout in the next vertical column, which contains a series of boxes divided by diagonal lines. In the appropriate box, write the resistance above the number of repetitions you complete in correct form. Carry your chart with you as you strength train.

ASAP STRENGTH-TRAINING ROUTINE						
Name:			Weeks:			
Date:						
Exercise Body Weight:						
1.						
2.						
3.						
4.						
5.						
6.						
7.						
8.						
9.						
10.						

12

ADAPTATION:
MODIFY THE PROGRAM

From working with thousands of overfat and out-of-shape people, I've heard almost all of the possible requests for adaptations to the ASAP program. For example:

"I'm a vegetarian. What should I do?"

"Can I skip the milk products?"

"What about switching the evening meal with lunch?"

"How about letting me trade a low-fat candy bar for the recommended snacks?"

"My local deli carries fresh bagels. Can I use them instead of the frozen brand?"

"Help, I've got to be at an important meeting at this great restaurant. What should I do?"

"I'd like to exercise on the equipment at the fitness center. Which machines should I use?"

I'm sympathetic to some requests, but to others, I'm not. It all depends on the nature of what's involved.

Let's discuss all these concerns and when and how to modify the ASAP program.

Vegetarian Meals

People who restrict or eliminate foods of animal origin from their diets are called vegetarians. The main reasons individuals choose vegetarian alternatives are because they believe it is healthier and more natural, they think it is more ecologically sound, or they adhere to religious or moral dictates that eliminate meat.

The vegetarians that I've worked with in the ASAP eating plan have all been knowledgeable in the food and nutrition area. Here are some ways that they adapt the basic menus:

- Sandwich and chef salad: instead of chicken or turkey, use tofu or black beans.
- Soup: instead of Healthy Choice Chicken Pasta, try Healthy Choice Garden Vegetable (220).
- Frozen microwavable meals: instead of Beef Tips, Glazed Chicken, Beef Stroganoff, and Roast Turkey, substitute the following from Lean Cuisine: Zucchini Lasagna (240), Marinara Twist (240), Three Bean Chili with Rice (210), and Angel Hair Pasta (210).

Milk and Digestive Problems

Some people can't completely digest the sugar in milk and milk products. This problem is called lactose intolerance and can lead to bloating, excessive gas, abdominal cramping, and diarrhea. Statistics reveal that lactose intolerance is prevalent in 8 percent of white Americans, 70 percent of African Americans, and 85 percent of Japanese. As individuals who have inherited this problem age, they gradually lose the ability to produce lactase, an enzyme that helps digest the lactose in milk and other dairy products.

Since the ASAP eating plan contains skim milk, yogurt, and cheese, how does someone who is lactose intolerant deal with these foods?

There are supermarket products that supply the enzyme lactase in pill or liquid form. Some of the brand names are Dairy Ease, Lactaid, Lactogest, and Lactrase. When consumed in the recommended dosages, any of these products can break down milk sugar and eliminate previous digestive problems.

Food Substitutions

Fresh bagel for frozen bagel. Though a fresh bagel is tasty, the problem is that most fresh bagels contain well over the allowed 210 calories of the frozen bagel. A 1996 report that analyzed bagels from more than a dozen New York bakers found that not one supplied less than 250 calories. Interestingly, some of the bagels were advertised as being low in calories, or less than 250. Many, in fact, actually supplied from 500 to 600 calories each. Stick to the recommended frozen bagels for breakfast. You can be sure of their calories.

Candy bar for fruit. No, fruit wins this comparison every time. Yes, I know there are indeed low-fat, high-fiber, nutritious candy bars that are now available. But there are also still plenty of candy bars that are loaded with calories. Don't tempt yourself by having candy bars of any type handy. Instead, keep your kitchen well stocked with whole fruit.

Diet Coke for water. No, don't substitute a diet Coke for water. A diet Coke supplies caffeine and some sodium. Even the caffeine-free versions have sodium. If you must have a diet soda, the one I recommend is Diet-Rite. It contains no calories, no caffeine, and no sodium—and it is available in many different flavors.

Apple juice for orange juice. Although orange juice is more nutrient rich than apple juice, you may use apple juice. A better substitution, however, is V-8 juice.

Salad dressing for light margarine. The Smart Beat Super Light Margarine, which I recommend, has two grams of fat and twenty calories in one serving. It is *not* a fat-free spread. You need the fat calories that it provides on your sandwich. But I also realize that some people would rather make a sandwich using some sort of mayonnaise. You may substitute a mayonnaise dressing if you can find one that contains two to three grams of fat and twenty-five to thirty calories for a one-tablespoon serving.

Lunch and dinner switch. Since all the ASAP lunch and dinner meals provide 300 calories, it's okay to switch them. In other words, you can have your dinner at lunchtime, or your lunch at dinnertime.

Other frozen microwavable evening meals. There are hundreds of frozen microwavable meals that are available today from a large supermarket. New brands and new versions of existing brands are introduced every week. Plus, many are low in fat, calories, and sodium—and are quite acceptable as far as taste goes. The problem is that many of these meals—especially the entrées with fish and seafood—are too low in fat. Remember, a good evening meal has approximately 20 percent of its calories from fat. Thus, a frozen microwavable meal with 250 calories should contain 50 calories of fat, or approximately 5.5 grams. Of course, if the calories from fat are two low, or too high, you can compensate by adding or subtracting fat from other foods and meals. Though I've done that on appropriate menus, it can become somewhat complicated. I want you to become an educated label reader, but unless you're really into nutritional analyses, my advice is to stay with the listed frozen microwavable meals. Do not try to mix and mingle them with others. Get your excessive body fat off first. Then you can consider some new choices.

Chewing gum. Several years ago if you'd have asked me about chewing gum, I'd have told you to forget it. Sipping cold water, I would have said, is a much better way to keep your mouth busy during the day. But Barry Ozer, who demonstrates some of the exercises in the last part of this chapter, changed my mind. He also lost 71¼ pounds of fat and 13¾ inches off his waist. Barry noted that the combination of chewing gum and sipping water really helped him concentrate better while he was studying for his MBA degree at the University of Florida. "The best gum," Barry said, "is Extra. I also like Care Free. Both contain five to eight calories per chew. Neither kind gets hard when it comes in contact with your ice water. I allowed myself up to five sticks per day, and I know it helped get me through a lot of temptations." Since then, I've recommended chewing gum to some participants—especially the ones who tended to be hyperactive. The majority of these people have found that chewing gum helped take some of the edge off dieting.

More Calories for a Large Man

Large is an adjective I use to classify a man who is six feet two inches or taller and weighs 250 pounds or more. A large man, because of his surface area and mass, requires approximately 300 more calories per day on the ASAP diet than does a smaller man.

There are many ways that a large man can add 300 calories per day to the basic eating plan. The way I recommend, however, is simple. First, you need to remember that after the Quick Start, or weeks one and two, all men up their calories by adding three slices of whole-wheat bread to their basic menus. Along the same lines, I want a large man to add four slices of whole-wheat bread, or 280 calories, starting on day one. And to these four slices of whole-wheat bread, I want him to smooth on one tablespoon of Smart Beat Super Light Margarine, or twenty calories more.

Whole-wheat bread is a nutritious food. One slice supplies seventy calories with a breakdown of 70 percent carbohydrates, 17 percent proteins, and 13 percent fats. Spread on twenty calories of Smart Beat, which amounts to two grams of fat, and the composition improves to 65 percent carbohydrates, 16 percent proteins, and 19 percent fats—very close to the ideal 60:20:20 ratio.

Thus, a large man begins weeks one and two at 1,600 calories a day. At the start of week three, he ups his calories by 200, with—that's right—three more slices of whole-wheat bread. So now he's eating seven slices a day—plus maybe two more, if he's having a sandwich for lunch.

Too much bread? No, not at all. In fact, a well-known study was done by Dr. Olaf Mickelsen of Michigan State University. For eight weeks, he fed sixteen obese (large) men twelve slices of bread daily—plus whatever else they wanted for meals and snacks. The average weight loss at the end of the study was 16.6 pounds per man. Perhaps most important, none of the men suffered from hunger pangs, nausea, or headaches—and all of them still liked bread at the finish of the diet.

But just in case you get a little bored with the whole-wheat bread after three or four weeks, you may try other types—such as rye, oat, or sourdough. Just make sure you read the labels and calculate the calories correctly.

Active Men

Some extremely active men, who do not weigh more than 250 pounds, also require three hundred extra calories a day. Often they are men who work outside in hard labor jobs, such as construction, loading and unloading, or plumbing. Other men who work two jobs a day may fall into this category. Or college students who follow hectic schedules may respond better with extra calories.

You'll probably know that you require more calories per day during the second week of the program. You'll feel very fatigued, have little energy, and the strength training will seem much too difficult. Compared to the first week, the second week will be a real drag.

Richard Bartfield experienced such a drag during the second week of the Quick Start.

Richard: "I Thrive on My Daily Bread"

"I thought I was going to fall apart," noted Richard Bartfield, a graduate student at the University of Florida. "Those wall squats and negative push-ups left me shaking all over. I had difficulty driving home after the first several workouts." Plus, Richard didn't have time to sleep off the fatigue. He was right in the middle of coping with his Ph.D. requirements in the School of Pharmacy.

I recommended that Richard add four slices of whole-wheat bread to the eating plan.

"That extra three hundred calories made a difference," Richard continued. "I had a big turnaround almost immediately in the way I felt. I began to be enthused by the exercise, rather than dread it.

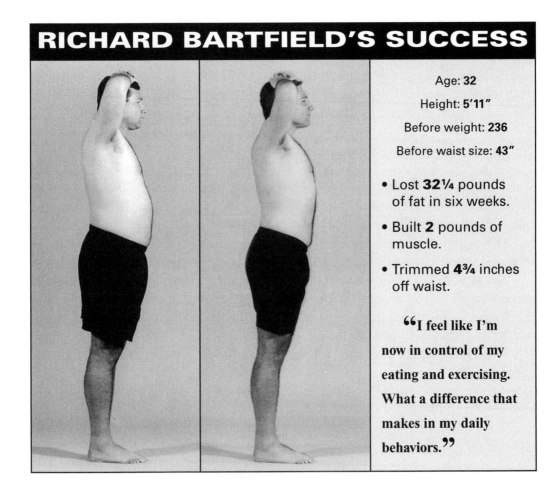

RICHARD BARTFIELD'S SUCCESS

Age: **32**

Height: **5'11"**

Before weight: **236**

Before waist size: **43"**

- Lost **32¼ pounds** of fat in six weeks.

- Built **2 pounds of muscle.**

- Trimmed **4¾ inches** off waist.

"I feel like I'm now in control of my eating and exercising. What a difference that makes in my daily behaviors."

"And all that bread—I thought I'd never be able to stomach seven or eight slices a day. Was I ever wrong. Now, I thrive on my daily bread.

"I've battled my weight for as long as I can remember. Both my parents were obese, which led to their premature deaths. As a result, I've read numerous books on weight loss and I've tried many, many diets. None of them worked very long.

"The bread, the simplicity of the eating and the water drinking, the slow strength training . . . at first glance, it all seems too good to be true. But it works!"

Less Than Six Weeks

What about a person who needs to lose only five to ten pounds of fat? How does such an individual modify the six-week program?

The original "10-Day Quick-Start Program" was designed for that purpose. In fact, numerous individuals who went through that phase accomplished their goal of losing five to ten pounds of fat and 2½ inches off their waist—quickly—in ten days!

You simply monitor closely your results at the end of ten days, two weeks, three weeks, or four weeks. If you are then satisfied, move directly into long-term maintenance—which is described in chapter 14.

But let me warn you, I rarely work with *any* man or woman who is satisfied—completely satisfied—with their results after two weeks, four weeks, or even six weeks.

So, even though you will reach your goal, you probably won't be completely satisfied. Maybe not ever. Such is human nature.

Eating Out on the ASAP Diet

I don't encourage my participants to eat in a restaurant during the ASAP program, at least not during the initial six weeks. It's simply too much of a temptation for many people to return to their old eating habits. At the same time, however, I realize that for some people eating out is unavoidable.

The absolute key concept that you must follow is to *be assertive*. You must announce to the managers of your favorite restaurants that you'll carry your business elsewhere unless they provide you with appropriate low-calorie foods. And you must mean what you say.

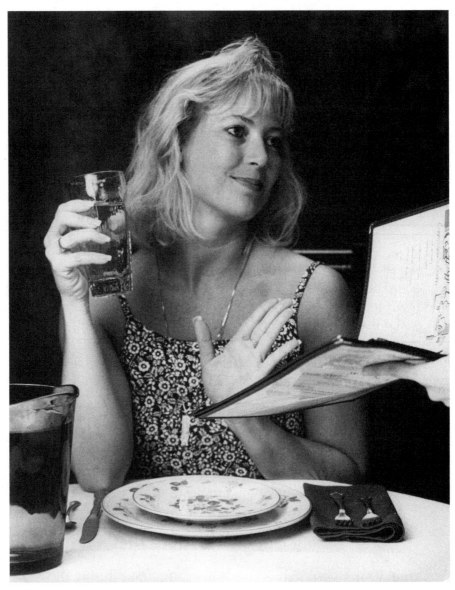

Put some discipline into your eating out. Ask for a pitcher of water, say *no thank you* to the menu, and order simply and assertively.

Here are the best rules to use when planning your meal:

- Request that a large pitcher of ice water be placed on your table. Drink freely before, during, and after the meal.
- Don't open the menu. The menu is supposed to entice you to spend big, and most restaurants know how to sell their rich, expensive entrees.
- Choose a simple green salad without such garnishes as croutons and bacon bits. Lemon juice, vinegar, or low-calorie dressing is preferable to any creamy or oily dressings.
- Select one or two vegetables with nothing added. A plain baked potato is nearly always available. Other good choices are broccoli, cauliflower, and carrots.
- Ask the waiter what kind of fresh fish is available. Order a white fish and have it baked, steamed, or broiled, with nothing on it.
- Be very specific with your order. Double-check to make certain that your waiter understands exactly what you want. Don't be afraid to send something back to the kitchen if it's not what you requested.
- Have decaffeinated coffee or tea for dessert, or at most, some fresh strawberries or raspberries.
- Reinforce the waiter and the manager as you leave. Make them aware of your specific likes and dislikes about the food and the service.

Strength Training with Machines

Millions of people in the United States have access to heavy-duty strength-training equipment. It's found in fitness centers, YMCAs, athletic clubs, universities, high schools, recreational centers, churches, hotels, and apartment complexes.

I'm very familiar with most of this equipment since I helped popularize the Nautilus machines that were best-sellers in the 1970s and 1980s. If such equipment is available to you, then it will be to your advantage to check it out.

Ideally, the facility should provide the following:

- A full line of strength-training machines, which includes exercises for the legs, torso, arms, and waist.
- Maintenance people who keep the equipment in good working condition. The upholstery should be clean and not ripped or excessively worn. The cables, chains, and belts should be tight and not loose or frayed. Plus, the workout area should be neat and clean.

- A staff of exercise instructors who answer your questions and help you organize and learn your strength-training routine.

If everything checks out to your satisfaction, then here's the strength-training routine that I recommend that you do for the next six weeks. The super-slow style, along with the other guidelines from the previous chapter, still apply. *Note:* In most commercial fitness centers, the equipment is arranged to be used in a specific order: legs, torso, arms, and waist. Thus, the ASAP routine is listed in this manner. If certain machines are not available, then substitutions can be made. Please ask an instructor for help.

The descriptions and illustrations that follow are for Nautilus and MedX machines. Other brands of equipment are similar, so the instructions should be adaptable. But regardless of the equipment or the exercise, work between four and eight repetitions. When you can do eight repetitions in perfect form, increase the resistance by 5 percent at the following workout.

MACHINE, ASAP STRENGTH-TRAINING ROUTINE		

Quick Start Weeks 1 and 2	Week 3	Week 4
1. Leg Extension	1. Leg Curl*	1. Leg Curl
2. Leg Press	2. Leg Extension	2. Leg Extension
3. Chest Press	3. Leg Press	3. Leg Press
4. Abdominal	4. Chest Press	4. Pullover*
5. Rotary Torso	5. Abdominal	5. Biceps Curl*
	6. Rotary Torso	6. Abdominal
		7. Rotary Torso

Week 5	Week 6	
1. Leg Curl	1. Leg Curl	
2. Leg Extension	2. Leg Extension	
3. Leg Press	3. Leg Press	
4. Lateral Raise*	4. Lateral Raise	
5. Pullover	5. Pullover	
6. Chest Press or Biceps Curl	6. Chest Press or Biceps Curl	
7. Abdominal	7. Abdominal	
8. Rotary Torso	8. Rotary Torso	
	9. Lower Back*	

*New exercise

Leg Extension Machine
(for front thighs)

Starting position. Sit in the machine. Place your shins behind the lower pads. Adjust the seat back against your buttocks. Fasten the belt across your hips. Keep your head and shoulders against the seat back. Grasp the handles lightly.

Movement. Try to lift the movement arm by only a barely perceptible ¼ inch. Proceed to straighten your legs slowly and smoothly once you start moving. Ease into the top position in approximately ten seconds. Pause briefly. Do not bounce in and out of the contracted position. Lower in a controlled manner in five seconds. Feel the weight stack touch, but do not rest or let the slack out of the system. Barely move again in the upward direction. Continue for the required repetitions.

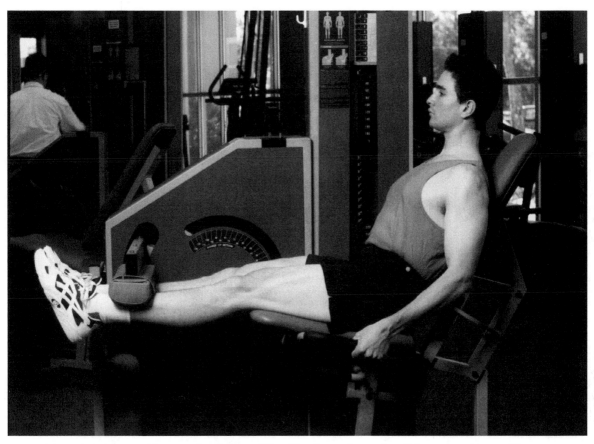

Leg extension machine, contracted position: Bend your legs smoothly as you descend the resistance back to the start.

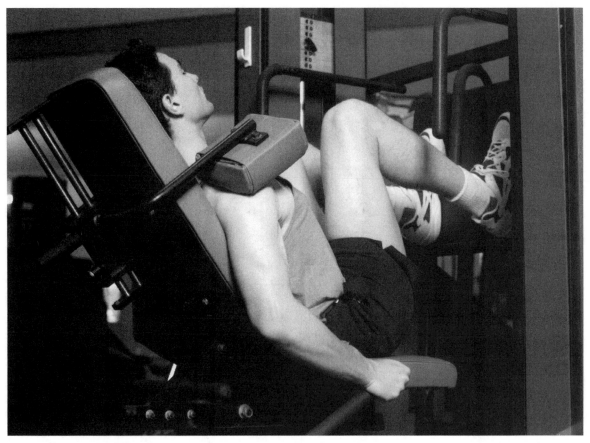

Leg press machine, starting position: Push with your feet and slowly straighten your knees.

Leg Press Machine
(for buttocks and thighs)

Starting position. Adjust the seat back and carriage to a comfortable setting until your knees—with your feet shoulder-width apart on the movement arm—are near your chest. The closer the seat is to the movement arm, the longer the range of motion and the harder the exercise. Note the seat position and adjust it to the same place each time you do the exercise. Grasp lightly the handles beside your hips.

Movement. Press with your feet and straighten your hips and knees in ten seconds. Do not lock your knees. Keep them slightly bent. Lower the weight in five seconds. Do not bang or bounce at the bottom. Smoothly begin another movement. Continue the lifting and lowering for the required repetitions.

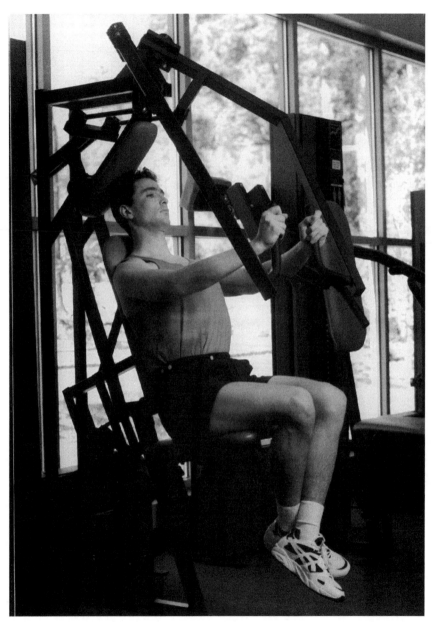

Chest press machine, contracted position: Avoid locking your elbows. Begin the lowering without resting.

Chest Press Machine
(for chest, shoulders, and back upper arms)

Starting position. Adjust the seat bottom and seat back to comfortable settings. You should be able to barely reach the handles beside your chest with your hands. Once these positions are established, note the numbers on the adjustment mechanisms. These numbers will allow you to duplicate the placements quickly during future workouts. Sit tall in the seat with your hips and shoulders stable. Grasp the handles by your chest and exert a little force to initiate the movement.

Movement. Press the handles forward slowly in ten seconds until your elbows are almost locked. Stop short of full extension. Reverse the process immediately. Bend your elbows smoothly and lower the handles beside your chest in five seconds. Repeat for the appropriate repetitions.

Abdominal Machine
(for midsection)

Starting position. Adjust the seat so your navel aligns with the red dot on the side of the machine. Fasten the seat belt across your hips. Cross your ankles. Place your elbows on the pads and grasp the handles lightly.

Movement. Expand your chest, pull gradually with your elbows, and shorten the distance between your breastbone and navel in ten seconds. Keep your shoulders against the seat back during the motion. Do not jut your chin forward. Do not pull excessively with your arms. Pull with your midsection. Pause in the contracted position. Return smoothly to the starting position in five seconds. Repeat for the required repetitions.

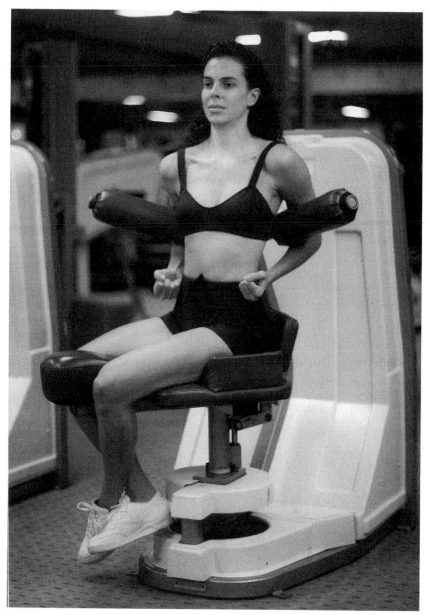

Rotary torso machine, starting position for left-to-right rotation: Twist your shoulders to the right slowly while keeping your hips and thighs fixed.

Leg Curl Machine
(for back thighs)

Starting position. Lie facedown on the machine. Place the backs of your ankles under the pad, with your knees just over the edge of the bench. Grasp the handles to keep your body from moving.

Movement. Curl both legs in ten seconds and try to touch your heels to your buttocks. Pause. Lower your legs in five seconds. Repeat for the required repetitions.

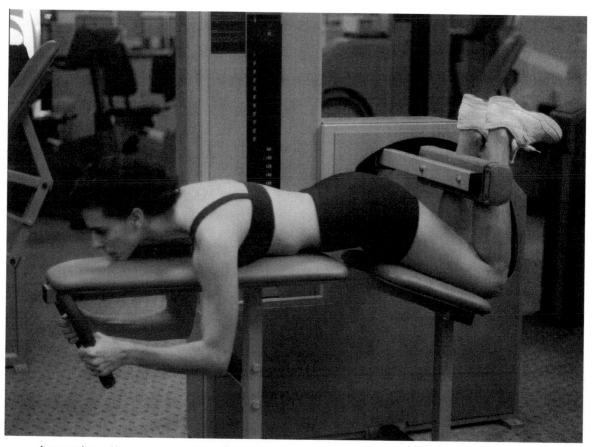

Leg curl machine, contracted position: Move out of the contraction smoothly and your hamstrings will be stimulated to become stronger.

Pullover Machine
(for upper back)

Starting position. Adjust the seat so the tops of your shoulders are parallel to the axes of rotation of the movement arms. Sit facing out and belt your hips securely in the seat. Leg press the foot pedals to bring the elbow pads forward. Raise both arms and place your elbows onto the pads. Grasp the handles with your hands. Release your feet gradually. The resistance on the movement arms is now on your upper arms. Move your upper arms backward into a comfortable stretch. This is your starting position.

Movement. Pull with your elbows and rotate the movement arms down. When your elbows are halfway down, lean forward slightly with your head and shoulders and continue to rotate the movement arms down and behind your torso. This entire 200-degree arc should take ten seconds. Pause in the bottom, contracted position. Reverse the process and smoothly allow your elbows to rotate up and backward into a comfortable stretch in five seconds. Repeat for the appropriate repetitions. On the final repetition, remove the resistance from your elbows by using the foot pedals.

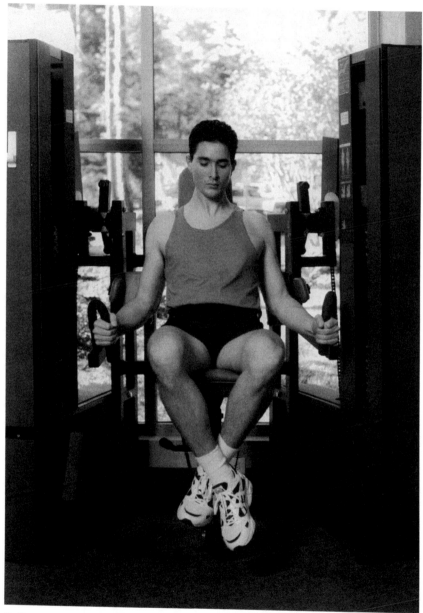

Pullover machine, contracted position: Rotate your elbows down and back at the bottom, and pause.

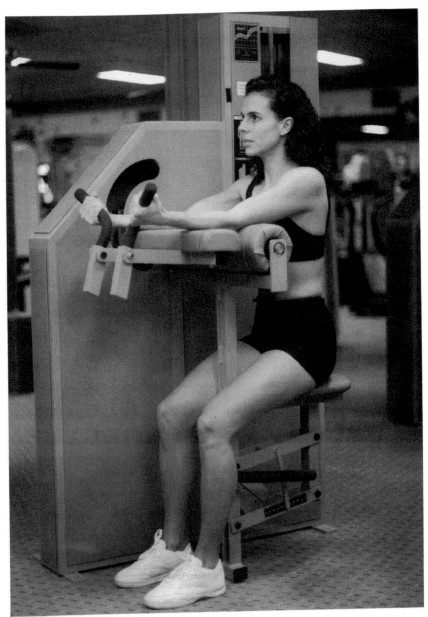

Biceps curl machine, starting position: Bend your elbows slowly and move the handles toward your shoulders.

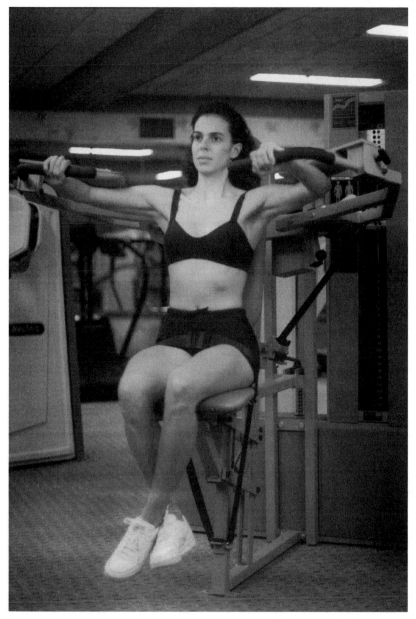

Lateral raise machine, contracted position: Practice keeping your elbows up and your shoulders down as you reach the top.

Lower-Back Machine
(for lower back)

If you have existing lower-back pain, or a past history of lower-back pain, consult with your physician before using this machine.

Starting position. Sit in the machine. Make sure your hips are well back in the seat. Adjust the footrest so your thighs are slightly elevated off the seat bottom. Some smaller men and women may require an extra pad to sit on. Fasten both seat belts securely across your hips and thighs. Put your hands across your waist and interlace your fingers.

Movement. Extend your torso backward slowly by rotating your lower back around the edge of the seat back. This entire motion should take ten seconds. Pause in the extended position. Return smoothly to the starting position in five seconds. Do not bounce or jerk in any phase of this exercise. Keep the movement under control at all times. Repeat for the required repetitions.

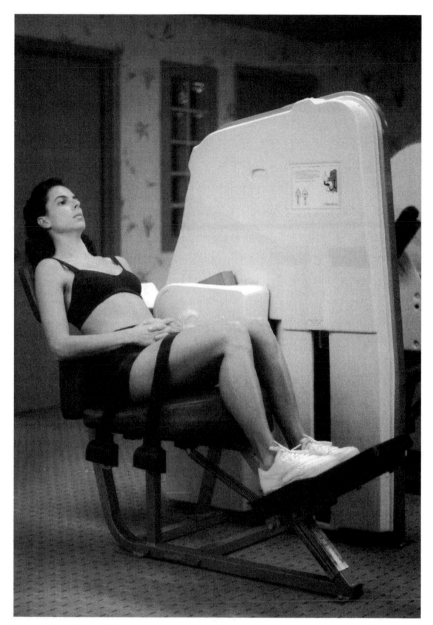

Lower-back machine, contracted position: Push on the platform with your feet as you extend your torso backward. Pause and release slowly.

Progress, See, Believe

As with the instructions from the last chapter, you'll want to make three photo-copies of the chart on page 128. List your exercises for each two-week segment in the first column. Then, in the next columns, keep a record of your workout-by-workout progression. Try to do one more repetition, or add 5 percent more resistance, each workout.

As your muscles get stronger, your stomach will get flatter.

Soon you'll see. Soon you'll be a believer.

ASAP

PERSISTENCE

Part Four

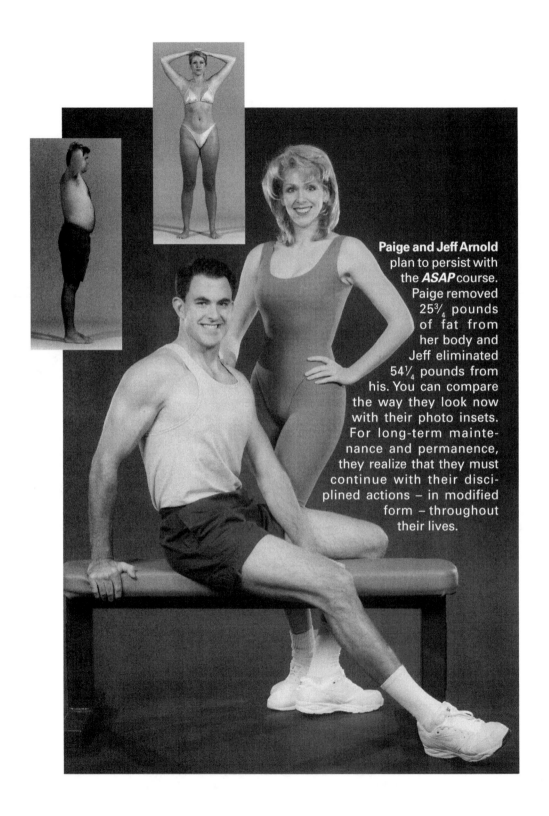

Paige and Jeff Arnold plan to persist with the *ASAP* course. Paige removed $25\frac{3}{4}$ pounds of fat from her body and Jeff eliminated $54\frac{1}{4}$ pounds from his. You can compare the way they look now with their photo insets. For long-term maintenance and permanence, they realize that they must continue with their disciplined actions – in modified form – throughout their lives.

13

PROGRESS:

CONTINUE THE COURSE

Six weeks equal forty-two days. Everyone knows that.

For all of you who have just completed the ASAP course, six weeks also equal most of the following:

- 47,600 dietary calories from 210 minimeals
- 8,064 ounces of superhydration from 63 gallons of ice-cold water
- 735 super-slow repetitions of 105 exercises from 18 strength-training sessions
- 52 miles of moderate walking
- 252 stomach vacuums
- 3,780 minutes of extra rest and sleep
- 714 visits to the toilet
- 588 other possible synergy-producing actions

Remember the old saying—*little things mean a lot?*

When you total all the little things above you start seeing the powerful effects that *A Flat Stomach ASAP* has on your body.

If you've applied the ASAP guidelines over the last six weeks, it's time to flip back to chapter 3 and retake your percentage of body fat and circumference measurements. Once you've finished, you'll want to compare your progress with the averages that I've compiled.

Inches and Pounds Lost

For comparison purposes, 41 men and 109 women went through the ASAP program under my supervision. Most of them completed the course in 1996 at the Gainesville Health & Fitness Center in Gainesville, Florida. The men had an average starting body weight of 208.3 pounds, a height of 5 feet 10½ inches, and an age of 36.3 years. The women had an average body weight of 156.5 pounds. Their average height was 5 feet 4 inches and their average age was 37.4 years.

Please examine the data in the chart below:

AVERAGE INCHES LOST		
Circumference Site	Men (N = 41)	Women (N = 109)
2 inches above navel	3⅝	3¾
Navel	4	3¼
2 inches below navel	3	3¼
Hips	2¼	2¼
Right thigh	1¾	2
Left thigh	1¾	2
Total inches lost	16⅜	16

If you look closely at the comparison data in the chart, you should see some slight differences between the men and women. Men had the greatest reduction (4 inches) at the navel level, while women eliminated the most (3¾ inches) at two inches above the navel. On their waists, women tended to lose from the top down, while men tended to shrink from the navel out. Both men and women averaged the same loss (2¼ inches) from their hips. But the women subtracted more (4 inches) from their thighs than did the men (3½ inches).

These findings reinforce the concept that men and women store and lose fat in slightly different places. But still, you can't help but see the overall similarities. Notice that the total inches lost were basically the same: men—16⅜ inches, and women—16 inches.

Don't be alarmed if any of your before-and-after differences are less than average. You can measure 20 percent lower and still fall within the normal range. On the other hand, if you have above average results, you should be elated.

How do these inches translate to pounds of weight and fat? Compare your results with the averages in the following chart:

AVERAGE WEIGHT AND FAT LOST			
Men (N = 41)	Before	After	Difference
Body weight	208.3	189.2	19.1
Percent body fat	27.3	17.9	9.4
Pounds of fat	56.9	33.8	23.1
Women (N = 109)			
Body weight	156.5	145.0	11.5
Percent body fat	33.7	26.1	7.7
Pounds of fat	52.7	37.8	14.94

Unless you had before-and-after skin fold tests done by an experienced tester, your percent body-fat calculations are probably going to be somewhat rough. I've had a lot of experience using the Lange Skinfold Caliper, and I applied it to all my research participants. Nevertheless, you'll still want to calculate your percent body fat and pounds of fat and compare your results with the average weight and fat loss from the chart.

The key numbers are in the *difference* column. The men lost an average of 19.1 pounds of body weight and the women lost 11.5 pounds. More important, both the men and the women significantly reduced their percent of body fat. As a result, both lost more fat than weight. On average, each man dropped 23.1 pounds and each woman shed 14.94 pounds of fat. Round off the numbers and they become 23 and 15 pounds respectively.

Simple division shows that the average man lost 0.55 pounds of fat each day and 3.83 pounds each week. The average woman lost 0.36 pounds of fat each day and 2.5 pounds each week.

If you accurately measured your body weight and percent body fat *before* and *after* the six-week ASAP program, your improvements should be near these numbers.

Muscle Added

Since the average man dropped 19 pounds of body weight and 23 pounds of fat, he must have built 4 pounds of muscle. That's an average muscle gain of 0.67 pounds per week for six weeks.

During the same time, the average woman decreased her weight by 11.5 pounds and her fat by 15 pounds. That means that she gained 3.5 pounds of muscle, or 0.58 pounds of muscle per week.

With hard work and attention to progression on all the recommended exercises, you should have added a similar amount of muscle to your body. Added muscle at this rate and level also means that you are significantly stronger—in your midsection, legs, torso, and arms.

In fact, this is the type of strength that is noticeable in photographs.

After Photographs

If you took full-body pictures of yourself in a bathing suit six weeks ago, you'll want to take them again. You should be able to see dramatic improvement when you compare your *before* and *after* photographs side by side. For valid comparisons, instruct your photo processor to make your *height* in both sets of pictures exactly the same. Carry this book with you to the store to help clarify what you mean.

Tammy and Joe: "We Needed Some Simple Rules"

"I would have never believed that I looked this fat," Joe Gentry said as he gazed at his before and after photos. "Look at my cheeks and my jaws—my face is the size of a beach ball. And check out my belly.

"Where's Tammy? Tammy, come and look at these," continued Joe in his amazement.

Tammy gave Joe a quick reflection. She was busy—busy examining her own comparative pictures.

Tammy, thirty-five, and Joe, thirty-six, were one of the many married couples that signed up for the ASAP course. Tammy is a commercial loan officer and the mother of two boys, ages eight and eleven. Joe is a computer salesman who travels frequently throughout the Southeast. Both had reached a time in their lives where their days were becoming more and more complex.

"We both needed some simple rules to follow," Tammy remembered, "and that's what this program provided. Do this, do that, and avoid these things. Joe and I respond well to specifics.

"It was a great experience for both of us to become involved in a joint project. So many times our jobs and responsibilities force us apart. But this course pushed us toward each other. We planned together, we shopped together, we cooked together, we ate together, and—we even worked out together."

Simple rules and togetherness—they clicked for Joe and Tammy.

Joe removed 40½ pounds of fat and 6¾ inches from his waist in twelve weeks. Furthermore, his beach ball face returned to "the way it looked when I first started high school."

Tammy also reduced and reshaped. She lost 3⅛ inches from her hips and 4⅞ inches off her thighs. Overall, she melted 23½ pounds of fat off her body.

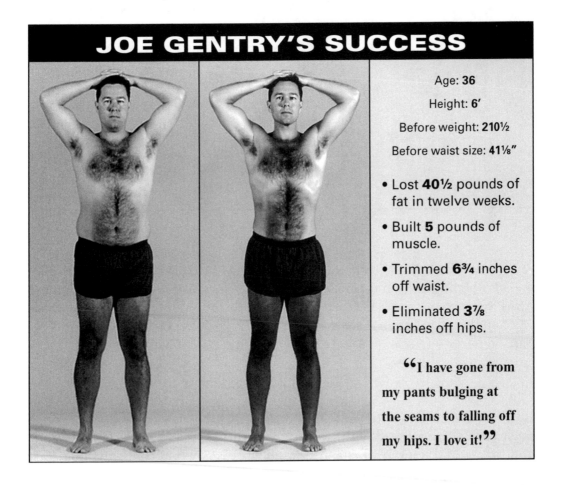

JOE GENTRY'S SUCCESS

Age: **36**

Height: **6'**

Before weight: **210½**

Before waist size: **41⅛"**

- Lost **40½** pounds of fat in twelve weeks.
- Built **5** pounds of muscle.
- Trimmed **6¾** inches off waist.
- Eliminated **3⅞** inches off hips.

"I have gone from my pants bulging at the seams to falling off my hips. I love it!"

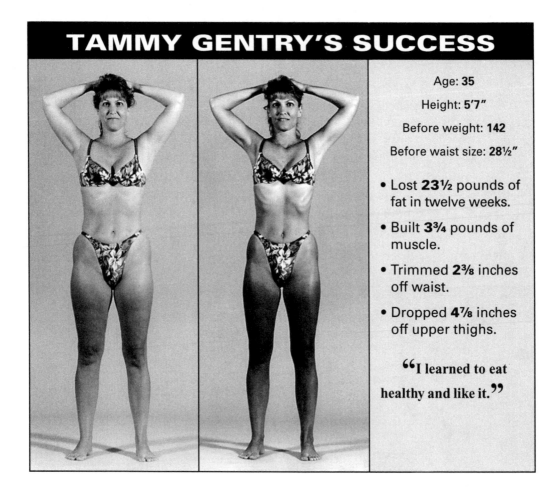

TAMMY GENTRY'S SUCCESS

Age: **35**

Height: **5′7″**

Before weight: **142**

Before waist size: **28½″**

- Lost **23½** pounds of fat in twelve weeks.
- Built **3¾** pounds of muscle.
- Trimmed **2⅜** inches off waist.
- Dropped **4⅞** inches off upper thighs.

"I learned to eat healthy and like it."

But it all solidified for both Joe and Tammy when they viewed their *before* and *after* photographs and realized just how far they had progressed during the ASAP course.

You should experience some of the same feelings as you examine your comparison photographs.

The Next Step

Have you reached most of your goals during the last six weeks? If you are like most people I've worked with, you still want to get rid of some more pounds and inches. The rest of this chapter shows you exactly how to do just that.

Commit Again

More than half of the people who finish the ASAP course decide to continue for another six weeks. With the same level of compliance, you should be able to get approximately 70 percent of the results. If you lost 15 pounds of fat during the first six weeks, for example, you'll lose 10½ pounds of fat over the second six weeks.

Make a commitment for another six weeks, or less if you believe you can reach your goal sooner. On the other hand, some individuals require three or four months or more to achieve their objectives. The key point is to decide now to turn your week-by-week dieting, strength training, superhydrating, and other practices into week-by-week steps that move you closer and closer to your goal.

Repeat the Basic ASAP Eating Plan

Six weeks ago, you began the eating plan with the Quick Start—which shocked your system into a fat-loss mode. For week three, you upped your calories by two hundred per day. Then, you descended your calories by a hundred per day per week during weeks four, five, and six. It's those last four weeks that now become your continuing ASAP eating plan.

In other words, eliminate weeks one and two, and concentrate on week three through week six.

The second time around you'll be more familiar with the menus and foods. You'll be able to judge serving sizes without actually weighing and measuring. You'll be more efficient with the entire system. Just be sure your daily calories remain at the appropriate level.

You can continue this down-up-down calorie plan for as long as six months, or until you achieve your fat-loss goal.

Combat Holiday Eating

If you continue with the ASAP eating plan long enough you'll soon have to deal with holidays. Holidays present a problem for dieters because the parties and celebrations abound with high-calorie foods.

But it doesn't have to be a problem that you can't effectively combat, if you learn a plan of attack. Here are four steps on how to take charge during holiday eating situations:

Plan ahead, eat ahead. If the festivity includes a meal, find out what is on the menu. If there are not enough good choices, eat at home. Budget one hundred to two hundred calories for a little grazing.

Limit alcohol consumption. Alcohol is calorie dense. It also tends to cloud your ability to forgo other high-calorie fare. Never drink alcohol to quench your thirst. Stick to water and ice with a twist of lemon or lime.

Say no gracefully. You can flatter the hostess by telling her how delicious a particular high-calorie food looks; then ask for the recipe.

Cut calories when not at holiday parties. During the most tempting occasions, trim a moderate amount from your normal meal schedule. Try to keep all your meals at three hundred calories or less.

Modify Your Strength Training

During week six of the ASAP strength-training routine, you performed one set of nine exercises during each of your workouts. You should continue with this same basic routine of nine exercises—with several possible modifications— three times per week until you lose your excess fat.

If you've been doing your strength training with heavy-duty machines, as described and illustrated in chapter 12, then no modifications are necessary. Continue what you've been doing. Anytime you perform eight repetitions on any specific exercise, add 5 percent more resistance to the weight stacks at the next workout. As I've noted previously, progression in repetitions and/or resistance is one of the key requirements for stimulating your muscles to grow larger and stronger.

With the at-home, strength-training routine, which is described in chapter 11, some important modifications must occur. Soon, if you haven't already, you will become too strong for the recommended exercises. You will be able to do more than eight repetitions, in perfect super-slow style, on most or all of the nine movements. Using your body weight as a major source of resistance— especially since your mass is getting smaller and smaller—is no longer adequate or practical. Even with a home abdominal machine, you will not be able to load enough resistance on the carriage of the machine. So what do you do? How do you make the basic exercises harder, so you can continue with the same system of progression?

There are three possible alternatives.

1. Do more repetitions than the recommended eight, or perform a second set of the same exercise. I don't suggest that you try either of these

modifications. More repetitions require more time under contraction of the involved muscles, and once you exceed two minutes, the chemistry changes to inhibit muscular-growth stimulation. Two sets are not a better solution. Two sets, especially if you are on a low-calorie diet, place too much stress on your recovery ability. So once again, you will inhibit muscular-growth stimulation.

2. Locate a facility that has the necessary strength-training machines, join the facility, and switch to a routine involving this equipment. This alternative may be your best bet.

3. Outfit your home gym with more equipment. The least you can get by with now is an adjustable barbell-dumbbell set, approximately two hundred pounds of assorted weight plates, a sturdy bench, and a pair of adjustable racks to support a heavy barbell for use in the bench press and the squat. If you have previous experience in training with barbells and dumbbells, then you might be able to purchase such equipment inexpensively by examining the classified ads in your local newspaper. Most sports and department stores also carry this type of equipment.

Okay, those are your three alternatives, and I don't recommend the first. The second is a good choice. Simply review the last half of chapter 12 and make the transition. The third alternative requires a bit more preparation.

Turn back to the week six, at-home routine on page 102. Exercises 1, trunk curl, and 2, trunk curl with a twist, can both be made harder by placing a weight plate (five or ten pounds) or dumbbell (fifteen pounds or more) across your chest. Exercise 6, reverse trunk curl, requires more resistance on your feet or ankles. This can be accomplished with special ankle weights that strap into place, or simply by using a rope or belt through a weight plate tied securely around your ankles. Exercises 7, 8, and 9 are already done with water bottles or dumbbells. As you get stronger, switch exclusively to dumbbells.

The remaining exercises—3, 4, and 5—merit more specific instructions. You'll substitute the following: side bend with dumbbell for side bend with hands over head, squat with barbell for wall squat, and bench press with barbell for negative push-up.

Here's the how-to for each new exercise:

Side Bend with Dumbbell
(for sides of waist)

Starting position. Grasp a dumbbell in your left hand and stand. Don't be afraid to use a moderately heavy dumbbell. These are strong muscles. Place your right hand on top of your head. Your feet should be shoulder-width apart.

Movement. Bend laterally to your left as far as possible in five seconds. At maximum stretch, try to reach even farther with your right arm and elbow. Return slowly to the top center position in ten seconds. Do not let your shoulders drift forward or backward. Do not hold your breath. Repeat the bending to your left side for the required repetitions. Switch the dumbbell to your right hand. Perform the motion to your right side in a similar manner for the same number of repetitions.

During your next training session, remember to work your right side before your left side. Continue this alternation.

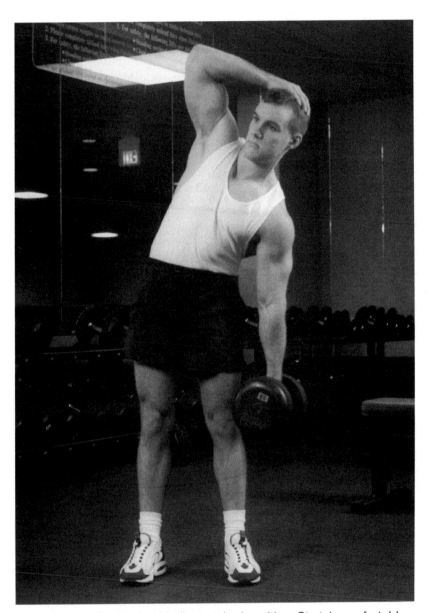

Side bend to left with dumbbell, stretched position: Stretch comfortably and return slowly to the top center position.

Squat with Barbell
(for lower back, buttocks, and thighs)

Starting position. Place a barbell on the squat rack and load it with the appropriate weight. Step under the barbell. Position the middle of the bar behind your neck and across your upper-back muscles and hold it in place with your hands. If the bar cuts into your skin, pad it lightly by wrapping a towel around the knurl. Straighten your legs to take the bar off the rack, and move back one step. Place your feet shoulder-width apart, toes angled slightly outward. Keep your upper-body muscles rigid and your torso upright.

Movement. Bend your hips and knees and descend smoothly in five seconds to a position where your hamstrings firmly come in contact with your calves. Without bouncing, and without stopping in the bottom, gradually make the turnaround from down to up. Lift the barbell slowly back to the top in ten seconds. Do not lock your knees. Keep a slight bend in them. Repeat for the required repetitions. As a safety measure during the squat, have two people act as spotters on each end of the barbell.

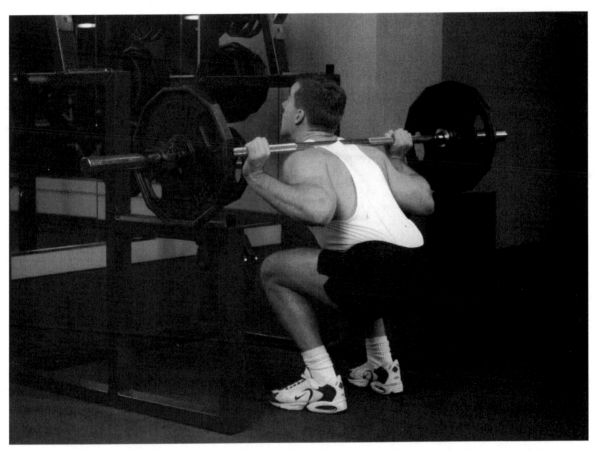

Squat with barbell, bottom position: Reverse the movement when your hamstrings come into firm contact with your calves. Keep your head up and progress slowly to the top.

Bench Press with Barbell
(for chest, shoulders, and back of upper arms)

Starting position. Place a barbell on the rack at the end of a flat exercise bench. Load the barbell with the appropriate weight. Lie on the bench with your shoulders under the barbell and your feet in a stable position on the floor. Grasp the barbell with your hands shoulder-width apart. Straighten your arms to bring the barbell directly above your shoulders.

Movement. Lower the barbell smoothly to your chest in five seconds. Barely touch your chest and reverse the motion inch by inch. Press the weight slowly to the top in ten seconds. Keep a slight bend in your elbows. Repeat for the required repetitions. As a safety measure, always have a spotter present.

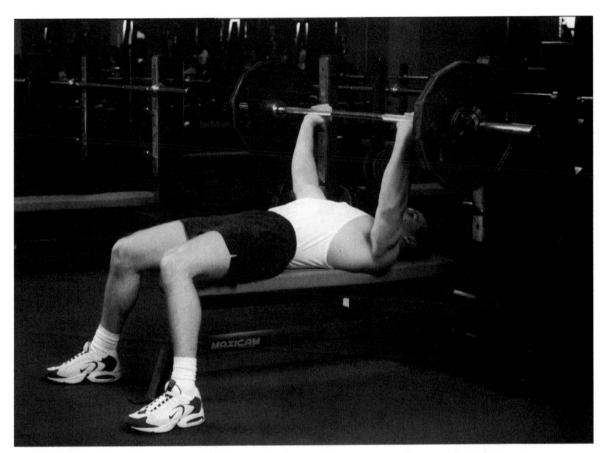

Bench press with barbell, starting position: Lower the barbell to your chest by bending your elbows.

Continue Other Practices

Along with your eating and strength training, your other practices—such as superhydrating, moderate walking, and extra resting—should remain at the same level as during week six.

Your goals, if they are on target, are only weeks away. Stay on course.

14

PATIENCE:

MAINTAIN YOUR RESULTS

atience is the ability to endure without complaint. It allows you to stick to a task until completion.

It takes patience to get your fat off, to strengthen your muscles, to flatten your stomach—and most important—to maintain those results permanently.

Patience, like any other virtue, must be learned. But how long does it take to become patient?

To help answer this question, I've gathered some related facts while working with thousands of overfat people, especially from observing the successful compared to the unsuccessful. From more than thirty years of study, the single most relevant fact that I've observed helps maintain results is *overlearning*.

Overlearning and Success

Overlearning means practice beyond goal achievement. Seldom does a serious-minded athlete ever practice enough. Larry Bird, the now retired all-pro basketball superstar, is sure that he shot the ball at the basket not thousands of times, not hundreds of thousands of times—but millions of times! Overlearning is one reason why Bird is such a superior shooter.

Overlearning, as it relates to *A Flat Stomach ASAP*, means the practicing of certain behaviors again and again until they are so ingrained that almost nothing can disturb them. Overlearning produces automatic actions. Without thinking, you respond with the correct behavior. The more times you experience the desired response, the better you get and the more lasting the pattern becomes.

Of the 98 people who successfully finished the original Nautilus diet plan in 1985, combined with the 150 people who completed the ASAP course in 1996, as well as thousands more who have been in my programs in between, the ones who have kept their fat off have done so because of overlearning. The salient rules—such as eat smaller meals, superhydrate your system, and keep your muscles strong—have been internalized.

How long does it take to overlearn and internalize?

A Hundred Days to Overlearning

I've observed with my participants that it takes approximately twenty-one days to establish a pattern and a hundred days to make that pattern automatic. In other words, the ASAP program gets easier for most people after three weeks. If they continue with the plan for three months, their daily actions become almost automatic.

Be aware, too, that many psychologists believe that the hundred-day time span means a hundred *consecutive* days. If you practice the discipline for forty-two days and break the pattern on day forty-three, then you must start over. Maybe that's why it's so hard for many people to keep the fat off permanently.

Yet I've seen many people succeed. One person who stands out in my mind is Barry Ozer.

Barry: In Control and Liking It

Barry Robert Ozer was in one of the initial groups that went through the ASAP course in early 1995. He was a leasing consultant in Gainesville, Florida. After I put Barry through his first strength-training session, two things were obvious to me. One, Barry had the biggest belly in the entire group. At a body weight of 239¼ pounds, his stomach measured 44⅜ inches at the navel. Two, Barry quickly mastered the super-slow style of doing repetitions in the very first workout.

At the end of three weeks it was obvious, once again, that Barry was really into the program. He'd lost at least a pound each day. During the initial six weeks, he dropped 32¾ pounds of fat. Then, he shed another 28 pounds over a second six weeks, and a final 10½ pounds during a third phase. In total, over eighteen weeks, Barry lost 71¼ pounds of fat and 13¾ inches off his waist.

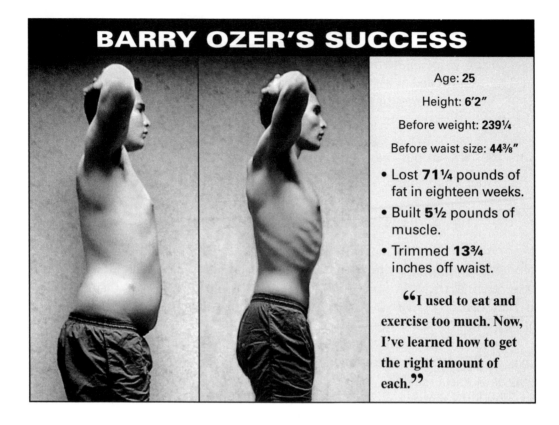

BARRY OZER'S SUCCESS

Age: **25**

Height: **6'2"**

Before weight: **239¼**

Before waist size: **44⅜"**

- Lost **71¼** pounds of fat in eighteen weeks.
- Built **5½** pounds of muscle.
- Trimmed **13¾** inches off waist.

"I used to eat and exercise too much. Now, I've learned how to get the right amount of each."

A lot of Barry's success was because of his discipline. "I kept track of everything with my calendar," Barry noted. "Each day I'd check off the meals, the water, the walk, and the workout. Before I went to bed each night, I'd put a big *X* through the day's date and mentally review what I was going to achieve tomorrow."

Amazingly, Barry showed me his calendar after I took his final measurements and photographs. From March 5, 1995, until July 18, 1995, it contained 135 *X*s—I know, I counted every one of them, twice!

How well did Barry comply to the recommended guidelines?

"One hundred percent," said Barry in his matter-of-fact tone of voice. "I didn't cheat a single time during those hundred and thirty-five days."

"Then, what happened?" I asked, curious as to what upset his discipline.

"I decided I wanted a piece of chocolate cake, so I had one," replied Barry. "And it was a big piece, too. But you know what? Halfway through that chocolate cake I knew I was in control—complete control. So I put my fork down . . . and ran straight to the toilet and threw up!

"No, I was just kidding," Barry laughed, which sort of made him seem even more real. "Actually, I just put the fork down, finished my glass of ice water, pushed back from the table, and went for my evening walk. Six months earlier, I would have probably eaten the whole cake.

"Since that day, I've had cake anytime I've wanted it. But the kicker is . . . I haven't wanted it very often. And when I do want it, I know how to compensate for it by cutting back somewhere else.

"The best thing is that I'm in charge now. It used to be the other way around: The food and the social environment dominated me. Not anymore.

"It feels great to be in control."

Practice and More Practice

Before Barry Ozer could say he was *in control,* however, he had to overlearn his daily rituals. In Barry's case, it took him 135 days—which is 30 percent longer than the 100 days I mentioned earlier. But remember also that Barry was very overfat. He had to lose more than 70 pounds of fat to reach his goal.

With most people who need to lose from 20 to 40 pounds, 100 days becomes an overlearning target. But my experience in dealing with thousands of people reveals that 200 days is better than 100. Within reason, more is better.

In fact, I just talked with Barry Ozer on the telephone, and it has been 500 days since he officially finished his three six-week courses. Barry says his condition is better than ever. You can judge for yourself by looking closely at the exercise pictures of him in chapter 12.

Maintenance Guidelines

Successful maintenance, like successful overlearning, requires a continuation of the practices that you've been adhering to for the last several months. There are, however, a few minor adjustments that you must understand and apply.

Follow a carbohydrate-rich moderate-calorie eating plan. Carbohydrate-rich meals are still what you should be consuming, but your total calories per day can be increased. Generally, a middle-aged man of average height and weight should be able to maintain his weight on from 1,800 to 2,400 calories a day. An average middle-aged woman would require 1,400 to 2,100 calories a day.

You can figure out your maintenance level by gradually adding calories back into your eating plan. A man should go to 1,800 calories a day. A woman should try 1,400 calories a day. Stay at this level for a week. If you are still losing weight, raise the level by 100 calories a day for the next week. In another

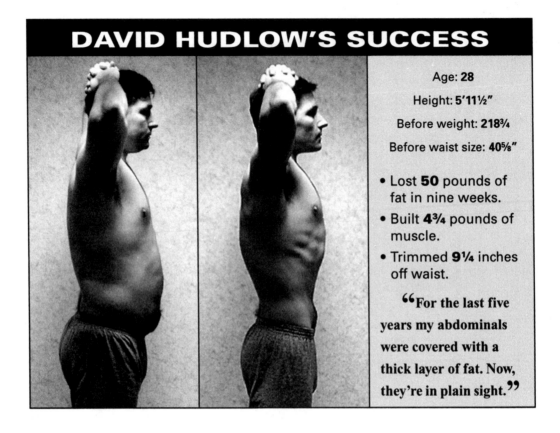

DAVID HUDLOW'S SUCCESS

Age: **28**

Height: **5'11½"**

Before weight: **218¾**

Before waist size: **40⅝"**

- Lost **50** pounds of fat in nine weeks.
- Built **4¾** pounds of muscle.
- Trimmed **9¼** inches off waist.

"For the last five years my abdominals were covered with a thick layer of fat. Now, they're in plain sight."

week or two, your body weight will stabilize. You'll then know that you've reached your upper limit of your maintenance calorie level.

Also you may want to turn back to the Simplified Food Guide on page 43 for suggestions on the 60:20:20 ratio of carbohydrates, proteins, and fats. Remember, fruits, vegetables, breads, and cereals are your primary sources of carbohydrates.

Eat smaller meals more frequently. You've been limiting your five minimeals per day to three hundred calories or less. To maintain your body weight, set the limit to four hundred calories for a woman and five hundred calories for a man. Sometimes a few extra calories per meal are acceptable. But anything more than six hundred calories in a meal means that your body will store the excess in your fat cells.

Superhydrate with at least one gallon of cold water each day. You've experienced the positive effects of sipping plenty of cold water. You should now understand the importance of superhydration in fat loss, muscle building, skin health, and internal and external cooling. Water supports your every function. Make super-hydration a permanent part of your new lifestyle.

Strength train twice a week. You must continue to strength train your newly built muscles, or they will shrink. Don't allow this wasting away to happen to your stronger, leaner body. Stronger muscles are one of your best insurance policies against regaining fat.

The primary difference between muscle maintenance and muscle building is that you don't need to train as often. Your frequency of training may be reduced from three to two times per week. Most people on my maintenance program work out on Mondays and Thursdays.

Keep in mind that more strength training is not better. Better strength training is *harder*. Apply this concept consistently, and your midsection muscularity and overall leanness may well exceed your goals.

Practice a few other actions, as needed. Any of the other actions—such as the stomach vacuum, moderate walking, extra sleep, and staying cool—can be reincorporated into your maintenance schedule anytime you may need a synergistic boost.

Back to Patience

A Flat Stomach ASAP: The Breakthrough Plan for the Look You Want in Just Six Weeks, the title and subtitle of this book, do not exactly stress the concept of patience. As you should realize by now, however, patience is an important aspect of the entire system.

The acronym in the title—ASAP—implies *as soon as possible.* But it also stands for the cornerstones of stomach flattening: Awareness, Science, Application, and Persistence. Each of these concepts requires patience to comprehend and incorporate all the recommended guidelines.

Persistence, the last section of this book, is the glue that keeps the system together. Patience, by the way, is often listed as a synonym for persistence.

Barry Ozer and the others whose success stories you've read about in this book have all learned plenty about patience in their personal journeys to flatten their stomachs.

As I said in the introduction, losing pounds and inches of fat from your waist requires discipline. The entire process demands *hard work.*

But because of the repeated hard work, it does, in a sense, get easier. It gets easier because the course teaches you to endure without complaint. And in the process, you perfect your patience.

Yes, patience is truly a virtue. And you've got it!

15

PERFECTION:

GO FOR YOUR PERSONAL-BEST ABS

Fifty years from now, historians may write about the latter half of the 1990s as being a time when people were obsessed with muscular midsections or great abs. Actually, this abdominal fascination is not new.

In 1953, I remember looking at the famous Charles Atlas advertisement for the first time. To the right of the comical drawings of Mac, the ninety-seven-pound weakling, his girlfriend, and the big bully at the beach, was a handsome picture of Atlas. Atlas was featured in a leopard skin swimsuit, smiling and contracting his abdominal muscles. That picture turned me into a bodybuilding fan, as it had many others who admired the ad before me.

But it wasn't until 1959 that I actually saw a bodybuilding contest. It took place at the downtown YMCA in Houston, Texas. One of the winners, Ed Cook, displayed the best abdominal muscles I'd ever seen. Four years later, while a student at Baylor University, I joined Ed's gym in Waco, Texas.

Ed and I trained together for five years. It was during that time that I sharpened my interest in anatomy, physiology, and strength training. We were both enthusiastic about our eating and exercising and we often traveled together to bodybuilding contests. Although I could match Ed in some body parts, I could never get my abdominals defined anywhere close to his. Ed Cook, like Charles Atlas, had great abs.

But as great as Ed's abs were, they weren't perfect. The abdominals closest to absolute perfection, in my opinion, belong to Frank Zane.

Frank, who is now well into his fifties, won the highest bodybuilding title in the world—Mr. Olympia—three consecutive years: 1977, 1978, and 1979.

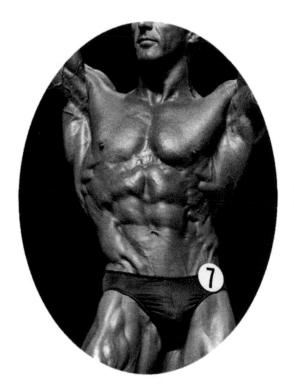

The muscular development and leanness of Frank Zane's midsection are superb.

Unlike the massive champions of today, who weigh 250 pounds or more, Zane never weighed more than 185 pounds when he was in top condition.

Frank was a master showman, and almost all of his poses revealed his midsection magic. His abdominals tied his upper body to his lower body very harmoniously. Frank overpowered his more massive opponents with symmetry. Symmetry, in Frank Zane's mind, began and ended with the abdominals.

"If you want to emphasize your abdominals," said Zane in a magazine interview, "train them first and last in your workout." Interestingly, that's the same advice that Ed Cook used to give the students in his gym. And that also happened to be one of the guidelines stressed by the Charles Atlas course.

Before I get into the exercise-by-exercise routine that I recommend for your quest for personal-best abs, I want to briefly cover a few salient considerations.

Not for Everyone

This chapter, or the application of the concept and routine described within it, is not for everyone. It is for those very few individuals who not only already have a flat stomach but are also close to having a concave formation running down the center of the midsection.

As I mentioned in chapter 1, achieving a concave stomach requires exceptional inherited traits or genes.

The Right Genetics

First, you have to possess the ability to achieve a very low level of body fat. A very low level of body fat means less than 5 percent for a man and less than 10 percent for a woman.

To give you an idea of how low those percentages are, I calculated percent body-fat numbers on each of the 150 people who started and finished the ASAP course. The starting and finishing averages for men were 27.3 percent and 17.9 percent. For women, the averages were 33.7 percent and 26.1 percent. These finishing numbers are a long way from the 5 percent and 10 percent levels that are necessary for success on the first aspect.

I have trained some individuals, however, who have achieved a fairly low percentage of body fat. Three of them are shown demonstrating the exercises in this chapter.

Stacey Ferrari, thirty-six, lost twelve pounds of fat in four weeks on the ASAP plan. She is shown in the hanging leg raise and the leg curl. At the time that the exercise pictures were taken, her body-fat level was 11.7 percent.

Craig Wilburn, twenty-four, was already in great shape when I met him, but he wanted to get better. I trained him for two weeks. He dropped 7½ pounds of fat and reduced his body fat to 4.6 percent.

Kerry Hamilton, twenty-four, had the lowest level of body fat of any woman on the ASAP plan. She registered 8.8 percent after losing 6 pounds in two weeks.

For comparison purposes, I'll list the body-fat percentage levels of the individuals pictured in the exercise shots in chapters 11 and 12—Paige Arnold: 17.1 percent; Jeff Arnold: 8 percent; Lisa Danver: 18.5 percent (see page 123); Ana Rocha: 16 percent (see page 147); and Barry Ozer: 7.6 percent.

Mike Derringer, who is featured on page 6, had the lowest level of body fat of any ASAP participant. After losing twelve pounds in two weeks, Mike measured 4.3 percent body fat. Jenny Rogers, pictured on the same page as Mike, had a body-fat level of 12.6 percent.

Remember in chapter 2, when I pointed out that fat cells inside the body can range from a low of 10 billion to a high of 250 billion? It is obvious to me that Stacey Ferrari, Craig Wilburn, Kerry Hamilton, Mike Derringer, and Jenny

Rogers have fat cell numbers that are on the low side of the range. Having a low number of fat cells is primarily genetic, since over 90 percent of your fat cells were already established prior to your birth.

A low number of fat cells allows you to get a small percentage of body fat. But that in itself is not enough for great abs.

Second, you must have a favorable ordering of the spots that you lose fat from. In other words, when you lose fat it must come off your midsection first or second and not last.

Most of the fat that an average person has is located between the skin and muscle all over the body. Thin layers are around the feet, hands, and head. The layers thicken toward the body's core. The upper arms and thighs, for example, have thicker layers than do the forearms and calves. The thickest layers of fat for a man are located on his waist, usually around the navel and over the sides between the lower ribs and pelvic girdle. A woman sometimes stores fat there, too, but usually her thickest layers are over the buttocks and upper thighs.

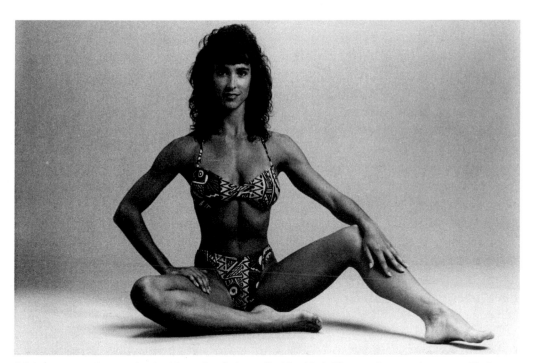

Of the women I've worked with at the Gainesville Health & Fitness Center, the one with the best combination of muscle, leanness, and midsection sharpness was Jill McCann. When this photograph was taken, Jill was 25 years old, 5 feet 6 inches tall, and weighed 127 pounds—with a body-fat level of 11.2 percent and a waist size of 24½ inches. Jill is also pictured on pages 53 and 80.

Fat deposition and fat reduction are ordered processes. A typical man might deposit fat first on the sides of his waist. Second, it might go over the navel area; then the hips and chest; then the upper arms and thighs; and finally the calves, forearms, hands, feet, and head. When he reduces fat, it comes off in reverse: first from the head, feet, hands, forearms, and calves; then the thighs and upper arms; followed by the chest and hips; and finally the navel area and sides. Once again, the ordering above is typical.

But there are a few people who have different orderings of where fat is stored. These people lose fat first or second from their waist. Rather than be a huge struggle, as it is for most of us, their waistline fat comes off moderately easily. So these few people have an advantage in the quest for exceptional abs. But once again, that advantage has little to do with eating or exercising. It's primarily genetic.

Third, once the fat is off the midsection, you still must have symmetrically paired, well-developed rectus abdominis muscles. Most people who are extremely lean in the midsection can display three paired rectangular blocks of muscle. These formations are often called six packs, even though some people have a fourth pair of blocks. These blocks are caused by tendinous intersections. An inch-wide strip of tendon, called the linea alba, runs vertically down the center of the waist. Then, three or four other tendons stretch horizontally and connect to the vertical tendon.

But as is often the case throughout the body, many times the left muscle blocks don't match the right muscle blocks. Sometimes the right muscle is thicker than the left. Or the tendons on the left side are not parallel to the right tendons. Or perhaps the tendons are wavy instead of straight.

In a bodybuilding contest, the judges usually prefer the symmetrical, evenly developed blocks with parallel tendons. Sometimes, as in Frank Zane's case, there's actually more interest created in adding a twist or tilt to a slight imperfection. Such is the magic of understanding symmetry.

So the highly sought after, symmetrical six-pack look for the rectus abdominis muscles is another characteristic that is genetic. The rare people who have inherited this characteristic, however, do have a distinct advantage.

The Paradox

Here's the paradox: The very few people who have all the right genetics have had it too easy. They have great abdominals in spite of their training, not because of it. They would have had well-above-average abdominals with absolutely no training of any kind. But because they were not able to recognize their own exceptional genetics, they felt that whatever dieting and exercising they did produced outstanding results. Thus, is it any wonder that these individuals latched on to highly promoted fad diets, quickie exercises, and easy claims?

On the other hand, typical people with average genetics—and this includes about 80 percent of the population—have to work very hard to get into decent shape. But after years and years of training, they will not have the same level of abdominal sharpness as do the people who have exceptional genetics and do only limited training or even have poor eating and exercising practices.

Genetics is almost everything when it comes to great abs.

If you've got the right genetics for outstanding abs, then you will have already achieved exceptional results from the six-week ASAP course. This new routine will carry you to the beyond-advanced level, and quickly.

If you have average or slightly above-average genetics, then you're certainly welcome to try this routine. I hope you do.

But let me warn you. It's going to take super abdominal and upper-body strength to perform some of the recommended exercises.

Let's preview the personal-best abs routine.

Personal-Best Abs Routine

Nine exercises make up the perfect-abs workout. Apply the same guidelines as you've previously used in your other strength-training routines.

**ASAP PERSONAL-BEST ABS ROUTINE
WITH MACHINES**

1. Hanging Leg Raise
2. Side Bend
3. Leg Curl
4. Leg Extension or Leg Press
5. Lateral Raise
6. Pullover
7. Arm Cross or Negative Dip
8. Full-Range Trunk Curl and Sit-Up
9. Negative Chin

If an exercise, such as the leg curl and leg extension, has been previously described, only an abbreviated version will be presented in this chapter. Please turn back to the listed page for a full description.

Hanging Leg Raise on Machine
(for midsection and front hips)

This movement will tax your abdominals and hips from the first repetition. In fact, if you can perform eight strict repetitions of this exercise now, then you probably don't need this routine. But don't be surprised if you have difficulty doing one repetition the correct way.

Starting position. Hang by your hands from an overhead bar. A parallel grip works best, but an overhanded grip works too. Your body should be straight, with your feet near the floor. Your goal is to bring your feet up to your hands.

Movement. Start raising your feet slowly toward your hands. Lean back with your head and shoulders as your legs are lifting. Bending at the knees makes the movement easier. Keeping the knees straight makes the movement harder. Try to reach the height of your hands with your feet in ten seconds. Reverse the direction of your feet and lower your legs to the starting position in five seconds. Complete a second repetition in the same style. If you can't do at least three repetitions, then here's a tip.

Instead of using the standard super-slow protocol: ten-second positive and five-second negative; switch the positive and negative counts: incorporate a five-second positive and a ten-second negative. Since you are stronger in the negative or lowering than you are in the positive or raising, you should be able to do three or more repetitions in this fashion.

Or, if this is still too difficult for you, have your partner stand to the side and assist you by lifting your legs to the top. Then it's your job to lower your legs slowly to the bottom. Repeat for as many repetitions as possible. In a week or two, you should be able to work your way back to applying the super-slow protocol.

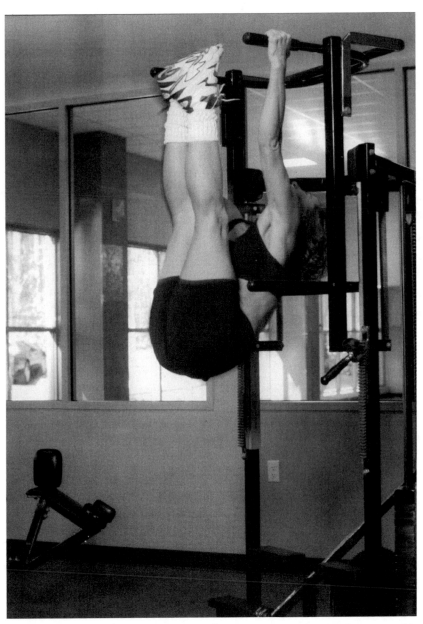

Hanging leg raise, top position: Pause briefly. Then lower your feet smoothly to the floor. Although this is a challenging exercise, keep practicing it.

Side Bend on Machine
(for sides of waist)

This exercise is best performed on the Nautilus multiexercise machine. Don't be afraid to use fifty pounds or more on this exercise.

Starting position. Attach a small handle to the movement arm of the multi-exercise machine. Grasp the handle in your left hand with your left shoulder facing the machine. Stand and place your right hand on top of your head.

Movement. Bend laterally to your left in five seconds. Return slowly to the standing position in ten seconds. Repeat for the required repetitions. Turn to your right side. Grasp the handle with your right hand and do the side bend in the same manner to your right side.

During your next training session, remember to work your right side before your left side. Continue this alternating process. When you can perform eight repetitions of the side bend to both sides in perfect form, add 5 percent more resistance and work upward again from four repetitions.

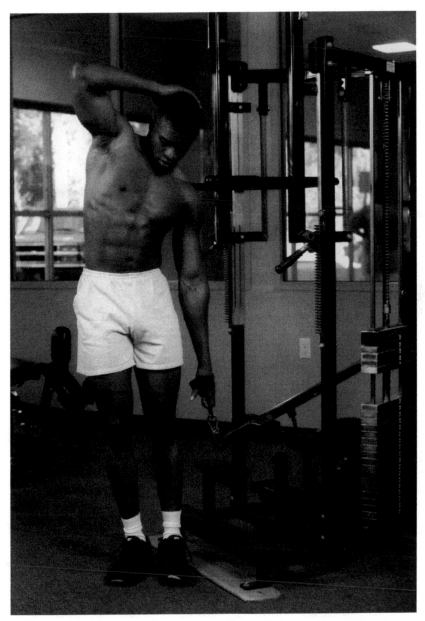

Side bend to left on multiexercise machine, stretched position: Be careful not to lean forward or backward. Stay in the lateral plane.

Leg Curl Machine
(for back thighs)

The leg curl was previously described on page 150.

Starting position. Lie facedown on the machine.

Movement. Curl both legs to your buttocks in ten seconds. Lower smoothly in five seconds. Repeat.

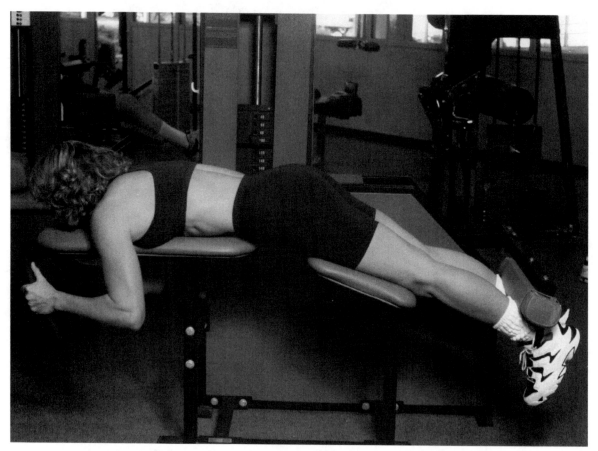

Leg curl machine, starting position: Keep your toes flexed toward your knees as you do this semicircular movement.

Leg Extension Machine
(for front thighs)

The leg extension was previously described on page 140.

Starting position. Sit in the machine with your shins behind the lower pads.

Movement. Straighten both legs slowly in ten seconds. Lower smoothly in five seconds. Repeat. The leg extension should be alternated with the leg press. Do not perform both on the same training day.

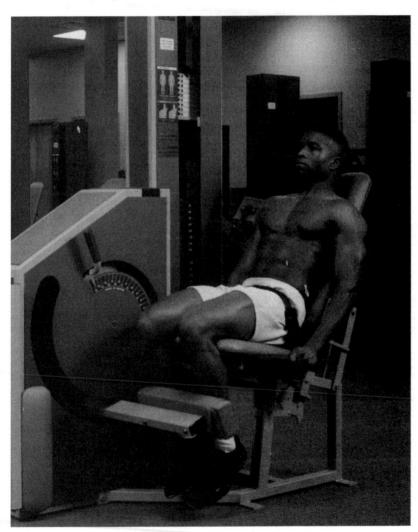

Leg extension machine, starting position: Stabilize your head and shoulders as you slowly start straightening your knees. After several correct repetitions, you'll experience a burn in your quadriceps muscles.

Leg Press Machine
(for buttocks and thighs)

The leg press was previously described on page 142.

Starting position. Adjust the seat to the correct position and be seated.

Movement. Leg press the resistance until your knees are almost straight in ten seconds. Lower to the starting position in five seconds. Repeat.

The leg press should be alternated with the leg extension. Do not perform both on the same training day.

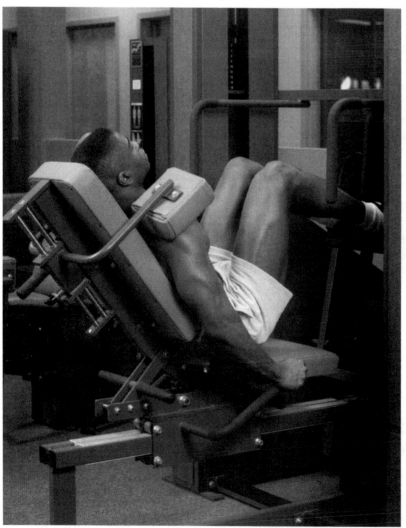

Leg press machine, starting position: Do the first several inches of the press very slowly, and your involved muscles will respond quickly.

Lateral Raise Machine
(for shoulders)

The lateral raise was previously described on page 156.

Starting position. Adjust the machine properly and be seated. Grasp the handles and pull back.

Movement. Raise your elbows slowly to ear level in ten seconds. Lower your elbows smoothly in five seconds. Repeat.

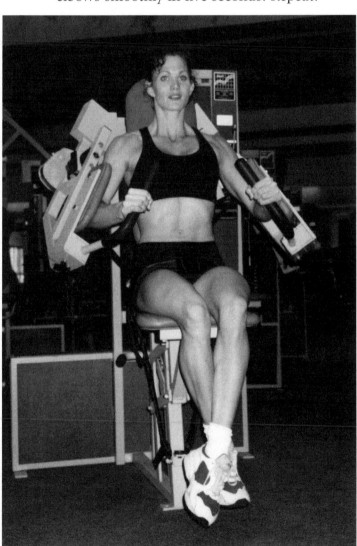

Lateral raise machine, starting position: Keep your head back and your chest forward as you begin lifting your arms.

Pullover Machine
(for upper back)

The pullover machine was previously described on page 152.

Starting position. Adjust the seat properly. Fasten the seat belt and situate your elbows on the pads.

Movement. Rotate your elbows forward and down slowly in ten seconds. Return to the stretched position in five seconds. Repeat.

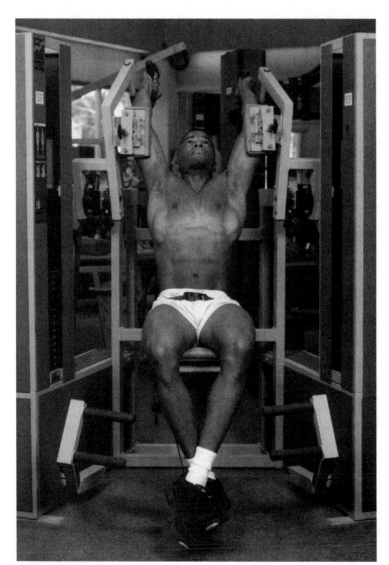

Pullover machine, stretched position: Relax your arms and stretch your upper back and shoulders. Gradually start pulling your elbows forward and down.

Arm Cross Machine
(for chest)

Starting position. Sit facing out in the machine. Place your forearms behind and firmly against the movement arm pads. Grasp the handles lightly with your thumbs under.

Movement. Push with forearms and try to touch elbows together in ten seconds. Pause. Lower the resistance smoothly for a stretch in five seconds. Repeat for the required repetitions.

The arm cross should be alternated with the negative dip. Do not perform both on the same training day.

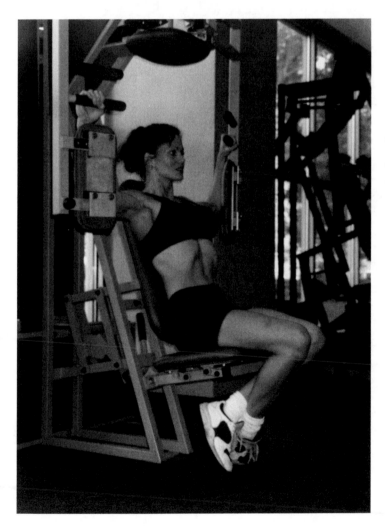

Arm cross machine, stretched position: Push slowly with your elbows and rotate your forearms in front of your chest.

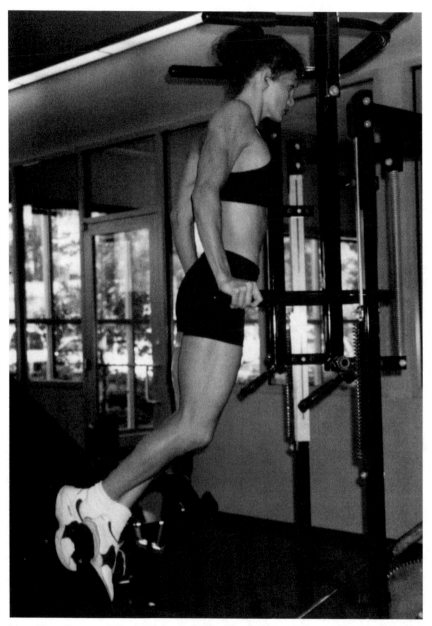

Negative dip on multiexercise machine, top position: Bend your arms and lower your shoulders toward your hands.

Negative Dip on Machine
(for chest, shoulders, and backs of upper arms)

The negative dip is best performed on the Nautilus multiexercise machine.

Starting position. Adjust the carriage to the proper level. It's important to allow ample stretch in the bottom position. Place your hands on top of the shoulder-high parallel bars. Climb the steps and straighten your arms. Lock your elbows and remove your feet from the steps. You should now be balanced and supported on your arms.

Movement. Bend your elbows and lower your body slowly in ten seconds. Lean forward slightly and stretch in the bottom position. Ease your feet on the floor. Climb back quickly with your legs to the top position. Lock your elbows. Continue the ten-second negative repetitions for the required number.

When you can perform eight repetitions in perfect form, step into the padded belt. Bend your knees and attach the metal ring to the movement arm's hook. You can perform the negative dip comfortably with a resistance attached to your hips. This is a very effective way to work your chest and arms.

The negative dip should be alternated with the arm cross. Do not perform both on the same day.

Full-Range Trunk Curl and Sit-Up on Steps
(for midsection and front hips)

Here's a superadvanced exercise that allows you to get a full stretch and a full contraction on your abdominal muscles. But it takes a little preparation, plus a partner to hold your legs in place. It's worth it though.

Picture yourself, from the side, doing a trunk curl. Move up to the contracted position. Now, lower your shoulders to the floor. But what if you could carve out a hole in the floor so your shoulders and head could extend below the surface? You'd get another thirty degrees or so range of movement for your abdominals as a result of this full stretch. With some creativity, you'll be able to rig up a situation where you don't have to ruin your floor in the process.

At home, you can perform the movement lying off the edge of an overstuffed chair or sofa. Your knees and calves have to be placed on top of the chair back. Your buttocks and lower back are on the seat bottom, and your shoulders and head extend off the edge of the seat cushion.

In a fitness center, you can do the same sort of thing by stacking the step platforms that are used by the group exercise classes. Here's how we do it in Gainesville.

Starting position. Assemble two levels of steps. The idea is to situate yourself where your buttocks and lower back, when lying supine, are about one foot off the floor. In my case, five of the stacked platforms are right for me. In front of the long platforms, assemble another much higher stack. Thirteen stacked platforms are perfect for my thigh length. Place a rubber mat over the bottom step to make the surface more comfortable on your back. Now, here's when you'll need a partner to help get your legs into the proper position.

Sit on the bottom platform. Lift one foot up and place the back of your calf on the top of the higher platform. Have your partner stand behind the higher platform and hold your foot and calf in a secure position. Do the same with your other foot and calf.

With both feet and calves now secure, test your seating. Check that your hips and thighs are in the proper position. Your thighs should be vertical and your hips should be flexed about ninety degrees.

Now, slowly extend your head and shoulders over the edge of the lower step. If your head easily touches the floor, then the bottom steps are too low. You'll have to add a platform or two to raise the height of the lower step, and you also have to raise the height of the higher step by the same number of platforms. As I said earlier, the numbers of platforms that work best for me are

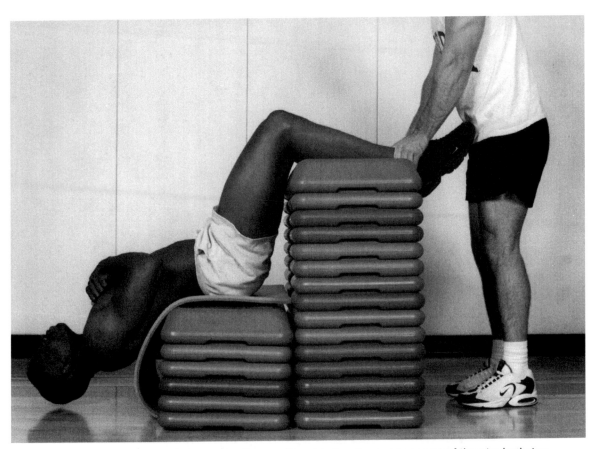

Full-range trunk curl and sit-up, starting position: Notice the arrangement of the stacked step platforms. Have someone securely hold your feet on top of the highest stack. Arch your middle back around the side of the lowest platform. Cross your hands on your chest. Extending your arms over your waist will make the movement easier, which most people will need to do at first. Remember, this is a very difficult exercise to do. Be careful getting into and out of the starting position.

five and thirteen. Your numbers may differ slightly, depending primarily on the length of your thighs and torso.

Okay, you're almost ready to begin the movement. Make sure all the platforms are interlocked and secure. Make sure you can extend your shoulders and head off the bottom platform. Make sure your partner knows to keep pressure on your feet and calves. Extend your arms over your navel and relax your shoulders and head and ease back into the stretched, starting position.

Movement. Curl your head and shoulders slowly off the bottom platform until you reach the contracted position of your abdominals. Your midback

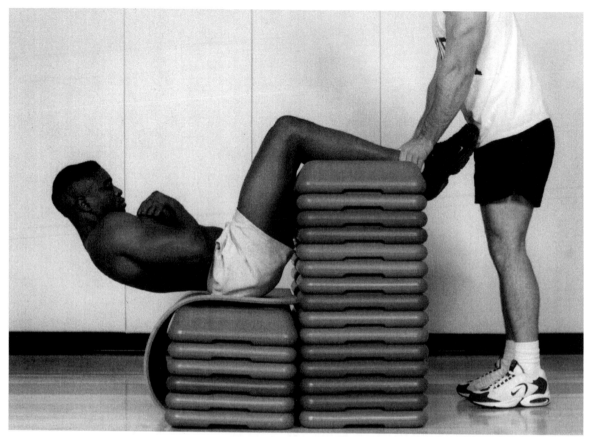

Full-range trunk curl and sit-up, midrange position: Roll your head, shoulders, and upper back forward slowly until your torso is slightly above parallel to the floor. This is the contracted position of your rectus abdominis. Now, the most difficult part follows.

should still be in contact with the bottom platform. But unlike the traditional trunk curl, where no one is holding your feet, your legs are now secure. Thus it's possible to continue to move forward—at least it is if you are strong enough in your abdominals and hip flexors. Continue the movement and try to touch your chest to your knees. Your arms should still be extended and on either side of your knees. Reverse the process smoothly. Lower your torso, shoulders, and head. When your middle back touches the bottom step, let your shoulders and head relax and extend over the edge for a comfortable stretch. Once you get the hang of this movement, your goal for each repetition is ten seconds up and five seconds down. But don't expect to do that at first. This is a very challenging movement.

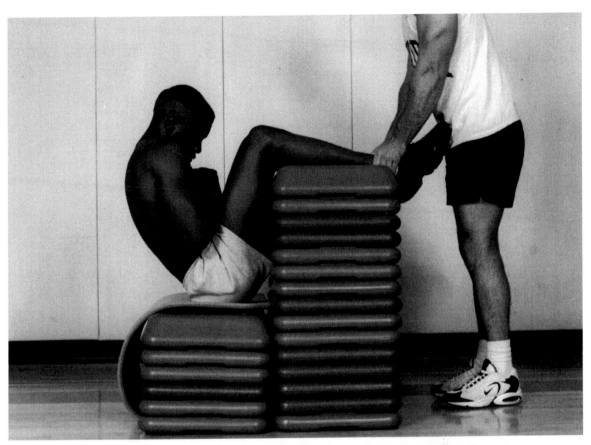

Full-range trunk curl and sit-up, contracted position: Use your hip flexors to pull your torso up and forward. Do the lifting smoothly and keep your chin tucked. Pause at the top. Lower to the starting position under control and stay focused.

You can make this exercise easier by placing your hands behind your hamstrings and pulling with your arms on the positive phase. Once you get up, release your hands and lower slowly. You can make this movement harder by moving your hands and arms back toward your head. I doubt if you'll ever need to place a weight plate across your chest for additional resistance. You'll be very pleased—I promise—if you can perform eight super-slow repetitions in the full-range trunk curl and sit-up.

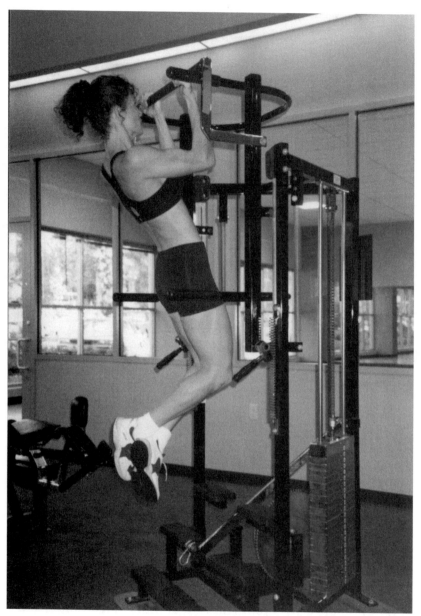

Negative chin on multiexercise machine, halfway-down position: Continue lowering your body by unbending your arms.

Negative Chin on Machine
(for upper back, front upper arms, and midsection)

This exercise, done immediately after the full-range trunk curl and sit-up, will add the final touch to your abdominals. You'll be using your arms to force your abdominals to a deeper level of fatigue. The negative chin is best performed on the Nautilus multiexercise machine.

Starting position. Adjust the carriage to the proper level. It's important to be able to get your chin easily over the crossbar when you are standing on the top step. Place the crossbar in the forward position. Grasp the crossbar with an underhanded grip. Your hands should be shoulder-width apart. Climb the steps until your chin is above the crossbar. Your elbows should be near your sides. Remove your feet from the steps, bend your knees, and hold your body stable with your chin over the crossbar.

Movement. Lower your body slowly, inch by inch, to a full hanging position in ten seconds. When you get halfway down, look up, arch your lower back, and force your knees backward. Try to stretch your body completely in the bottom hanging position before you make contact with the floor. Ease your feet on the floor. Climb back quickly with your legs to the top position with your chin over the crossbar. Continue the ten-second negative repetitions for the required number.

When you can perform eight repetitions with your body weight in perfect form, you'll need to add resistance to your body with a padded belt. Adjust the belt around your waist. Bend your knees and attach the metal ring to the hook on the movement arm. The movement arm is between the steps, and it connects to a weight stack. It is now easy to do the negative chin with resistance attached to your waist.

Some of my advanced male trainees have worked up to the level where they can do eight repetitions with a hundred pounds attached to the belt. Women have done seventy pounds. Use these poundages as a goal.

Your Best Effort

That's it for the advanced routine: one set of each of nine exercises performed in the super-slow style until muscular fatigue. Don't make the mistake of training your abdominals more frequently than three times a week or with more repetitions than your other muscles. Remember, spot reduction of body fat is not possible.

If you still have too much fat around your waistline, then you probably also have too much fat over the rest of your body. Keep adhering to the basic ASAP eating plan, the superhydration schedule, and the other related practices to reduce your percentage of body fat.

Frank Zane, the embodiment of near perfection, didn't produce his level of development overnight. Neither will you.

Give the personal-best abs routine your best effort for at least six weeks.

Who knows? A close-up of your abdominals may be the ultimate example and a perfect way to end this chapter.

16

PROBLEMS:

ADDRESS MAJOR QUESTIONS

In this book I've covered a multitude of topics, some only briefly. This opens the door for misunderstandings, which are usually followed by problems.

Problems generate questions, answers, and more questions. This chapter addresses many of those concerns.

False Hunger

Q. During the two-week Quick Start, I feel hungry sometimes. What can I do to fight the hunger?

A. You're not experiencing true hunger. True hunger occurs from severe deprivation of food. You'd have to be in a starving condition for many weeks or even months to reach such a state. What you're suffering from is false hunger, or your appetite is simply getting your attention. Remember from chapter 2, when I described the appetite-controlling mechanism in your brain?

There are several things you can do to keep your appetite in check. First, don't go longer than three hours between minimeals. Carbohydrate-rich foods trigger the right signals to your brain. Second, get up and move around. Being active raises your internal temperature, which also helps. Third, instead of drinking cold water, try a cup of hot decaffeinated tea. Hot fluids in your stomach will curb your appetite temporarily.

Urge Surfing

Q. What about just thinking to myself that I'm not hungry? Will that help?

A. Perhaps it will. In fact, I'm reminded of psychological studies that were done at the University of Washington by Dr. G. Alan Marlett and Dr. Judith Gordon. During these studies, they coined the term "urge surfing." The urge to eat, they found, is like an ocean wave. It formulates slowly, picks up momentum, comes to a crest, breaks, and subsides gently on the shore.

You might think urges come on like monsters that can be satisfied only by giving in, by submission, by eating. Caving into an urge results in more urges, more often, with more inertia behind them. But if you ride the wave, if you let it crest and pass, it will weaken and splash onto shore. Soon you'll become an experienced urge surfer.

There will always be urges associated with eating—the urge for a second helping, a salty snack, or a sweet dessert. The waves roll in most furiously during high tide, which translates to your high-risk situations.

Being a successful urge surfer means that you can detect the oncoming wave in time to prepare for it. You then have to be able to ride it out. Both of these—seeing it coming and knowing how to get on top—make you a good urge surfer. One without the other results in a lot of wipeouts.

Figure out your high-tide times by making a list of your high-risk situations.

Are you at high risk when in the house alone, maybe just before the kids come home from school? Or is it at night in front of the TV, subjected to an advertising industry unsurpassed at urging you to consume food? Are you a stress eater, using calories to douse the flames of frustration? Do you cope with boredom by pampering yourself with food?

Yes, you can learn to ride these waves mentally, or you can do it physically by substituting the three things I mentioned in the previous answer. Why not become skilled in both aspects?

An Occasional Dessert

Q. I know you don't permit desserts on the ASAP eating plan. What about the maintenance plan? Can I have a dessert occasionally on it?

A. Sure. The key is planning for a dessert and, most important, knowing how to compensate once you've consumed it. Just as Barry Ozer noted in chapter 14, *you* must be in control of the dessert—not the other way around.

If someone absolutely forced you to have a dessert several times a day, what would be your healthiest approach? Eat your dessert first, not last, in the meal. If you did so in a leisurely fashion, by the time you got to your main entrée, the appetite control center in your brain would already be receiving satiation signals. Thus, you might end up skipping some calories because you didn't finish the meal.

Perfect Score™ Shakes

Q. I've tried your Perfect Score shakes, and they're great. How did you come up with the idea for them?

A. In 1988, while director of research for Nautilus Sports/Medical Industries, I began experimenting with liquid meal replacements for some of my groups. I tested the effects of substituting one, two, or three meals with a shake that had from two hundred to three hundred calories. One or two meals per day worked better than three meals. Most participants also preferred consuming a shake best at breakfast, and then second at lunch. Few of them liked the idea of trading it for an evening meal.

The one thing that most participants agreed on was that they didn't care for the taste of any of the meal replacements. They all had a chalky, artificial taste.

When I relocated my office to Gainesville, Florida, in 1991, I continued to explore various meal replacements. One in particular, which was designed by a professor at the University of Florida School of Medicine, had a much better than usual taste. The reason, according to the professor, was that it used real milk protein in the formula.

Even though I applied this product successfully in several of my research projects, it did not contain my ideal blend of carbohydrates, fats, and proteins. As a consequence, I would have my participants add certain nutrients—primarily fat—to other meals throughout the day.

Finally, in 1997, Tim Patterson and I (we are partners in Living Longer Stronger, a corporation in Colorado Springs) decided to develop our own meal replacement. Our goals were to:

- Achieve my ideal macronutrient breakdown of 60 percent carbohydrates, 20 percent fats, and 20 percent proteins.
- Enrich the formula with appropriate vitamins and minerals.
- Use real milk protein and high-quality flavors to produce a superior taste and aroma.
- Render it into a powder that mixes easily with cold water.

I believe we accomplished all our goals. That's why we named the product Perfect Score.

Furthermore, in our initial testings we found that consuming several servings a day of Perfect Score contributed greatly to *metabolic equilibrium*. Metabolic equilibrium is a condition in which hunger is all but absent and mood is on an even keel. Such a state, we discovered, facilitates the entire process of losing fat and building muscle.

You must really experience Perfect Score and its effect on your metabolic equilibrium to appreciate what I'm talking about. And I hope you will.

You may order a box of Perfect Score, which contains thirty individual packets, by following the instructions on the last page of this book.

Homemade Shake

Q. *To get good results from the ASAP program, do I have to purchase a box of Perfect Score from you?*

A. No. But sooner or later, I hope you'll give it a fair trial. I believe you'll find it better than any meal-replacement product on the market.

In the meantime, here's a homemade substitute for the minimeal:

BANANA MALT MINIMEAL

Ingredients
8 ounces 2% milk
1 medium banana
1 egg white, cooked
1 tablespoon malted milk powder
1 teaspoon honey or brown sugar
¼ teaspoon vanilla
Dash of cinnamon or nutmeg

Combine all ingredients in a blender. Cover and blend on medium speed until smooth. It makes a nutritious and tasty minimeal of approximately 300 calories. Instead of the banana, you may substitute 100 calories of various fruits—such as strawberries, pineapple, or peaches.

And don't forget, you can always stick to the standard ASAP breakfast and lunch selections—such as the bagel, sandwich, or soup.

Festive Eating

Q. *The holiday season is approaching and I fear regaining some of my lost fat. What can I do to avoid all these festive calories?*

A. You're already headed in the right direction by being aware of the situation. And you're right, the average adult in the United States gains approximately seven pounds between Thanksgiving and January second.

Consider incorporating all of the following actions:

- Be conscious more than ever of the value of superhydration. One gallon of ice-cold water each day, at the very least, will work wonders.
- Take thirty-minute afterdinner walks regularly (get up and get out quickly—you'll eat less).
- Cut up a relish tray (or buy one from a deli) for snacks. Use nonfat yogurt for dip.
- Locate a nutritious vegetable soup recipe. Make a big pot and freeze in one- or two-serving plastic bags that can be thawed quickly.
- Rediscover whole-wheat bread (as well as other whole-grain products) and eat more of it. Remember, an average slice of whole-wheat bread contains seventy calories or less, and it's a real nutritional powerhouse.
- Stock up on fresh fruit in lieu of cookies, chips, and ice cream.
- Perfect a couple of low-calorie delicacies to take to parties. Use a magazine or cookbook that provides total calories, plus breakdowns of carbohydrates, proteins, and fats. Select one that has three hundred calories or less per serving and less than 30 percent fat.
- Eliminate alcohol altogether. Besides the waistline savings, you'll drive home safer.
- Say *no* to others urging you to eat against your will.
- Try to plan activities that are outings instead of just eatings.
- Practice staying cool. Dress lighter than normal. Avoid wearing a hat.
- Buy a tight-fitting New Year's Eve outfit, and try it on twice a week.
- Keep portions under control by incorporating nutritious microwavable dinners into your regular meal rotation.

- Give your low-calorie dinners the trappings of elegance—good china, candlelight, and soft music.
- Develop at-home strength-training equipment—such as water jugs or dumbbells—and use them if you're too busy to go to the fitness center.
- Follow up by keeping a daily journal relating to eating, superhydrating, and strength training.

The gist of this action plan is that you be strict about your calorie intake whenever you're not involved in a social gathering, and sensible when you are at them.

You're going to eat some high-calorie foods—in fact, *plan* on it. Neither forbid nor punish yourself. To enjoy this liberty and not pile on additional pounds, however, you have to counterbalance with moderate intakes at other times.

A frequent Perfect Score shake can be a time-saver as well as a nutritional boost. Remember, you need something in your stomach every three hours during the day.

Though you can pick and choose the suggestions you like, the most important thing is: Don't just cut loose; do not cast discipline to the wind. The seven-pound price you pay later will not be worth it.

Backsliding Forward

Q. I messed up on the ASAP eating plan over the holidays. In fact, I think I put back a few pounds. Help! What should I do?

A. You move forward, immediately. You're only human, right? Expect to backslide—not frequently but once in a while.

There is no disgrace in backsliding. The disgrace lies in letting a lapse get you so discouraged that you quit trying. Don't let yourself fall into this destructive trap.

True control and true power revolve around the realization that permanent fat loss is a long-term project that is bound to have ups and downs. You're feeling down now. Get up and move forward.

Favorite Family Recipes

Q. The frozen microwavable dinners have been a blessing for me. But after six weeks, my entire family wants me to return to all our favorite recipes. I'm afraid because I know many of them are loaded with calories. What should I do?

A. Food science research shows that the typical American family tends to eat from the same ten recipes repeatedly. Thus the development of ten leaner recipes is a management task for you.

Challenge every ingredient, one by one. Skim milk, not whole. Two egg whites instead of an entire egg. Ground turkey in place of ground beef.

Seasonings such as onion, garlic, and herbs, as well as some tomato and green pepper, will spice up ground turkey or chicken so you won't miss ground beef.

Replace sour cream in dips and toppings with a cup of low-fat cottage cheese whirled in a blender with one tablespoon of fresh lemon juice. Plain low-fat yogurt or buttermilk can be substituted for sour cream in salad dressings and baked goods.

Buy reduced-calorie light mayonnaise, or make your own with half mayonnaise and half low-fat yogurt.

Make soups and stews a day in advance so you can chill and remove fat before reheating and serving.

Cut gravy calories by using arrowroot, cornstarch, or flour to thicken pan drippings. This is in lieu of roux.

And don't forget about using nonstick skillets, or vegetable oil cooking spray, instead of traditional pan frying.

This sprinkling of suggestions and substitutions is only a start. Don't forget, calories do count.

Developing ten lean recipes based on your established family favorites is well worth the effort.

The Fun's Gone

Q. The ASAP program and the results I've noticed have turned me on to strength training. But now that I've finished the course, the strength-training exercise is not very enjoyable anymore. I used to have a lot of fun doing aerobics classes. Can I start doing them again?

A. Before I answer your question, let's go back a minute and define some concepts. Remember from chapter 5, I defined strength training as movement against resistance? Well—quantity movement against quality resistance, which is what's going on in the super-slow style that I recommend in this book—is certainly not fun. In fact, it's brutally intense when it's done properly. And that's exactly why such strength training is so productive for your body.

Aerobic- or dance-type movements to music, which are offered in many fitness centers, can be great fun. But there's a huge misconception in this country that all exercise should be fun. The reasoning is that if it is not fun, you won't stick with it.

Hogwash! If you're interested in getting *results* from your exercise—and that should be your primary goal: changing your body—then the exercise better *not* be fun. Having fun, I've found, is a sure way to stay overfat.

Edward Jackowski, author of *Hold It! You're Exercising Wrong,* interviewed a thousand women who were enthusiastically involved with aerobics. During the interview, he asked each one, "How many women, including yourself, do you know who have ever vastly improved their body by taking aerobic classes?"

All of them had the same response: "Zero." No one woman had ever either lost a significant amount of fat or built much muscle from aerobics. Yet most of these women kept returning day after day and week after week in hope that something would happen. They twisted, they turned, they stepped, they swayed, and they sweated—but nothing happened.

Why? The women who did aerobics received poor results because the exercise movements lacked intensity. They were not hard enough, slow enough, or progressive enough to produce growth stimulation.

"Do not take any aerobics class," Jackowski concludes, "with the expectation that you are actually going to change your body—because you won't. Take them because you enjoy exercising with others. Take them for fun."

I agree with Jackowski's findings. Even under the best conditions, an aerobics class is not an efficient way to lose fat or build muscle. But it sure is fun.

On the other hand, proper strength-training exercise is grueling. There's no question about it. Few of my ASAP participants have ever really liked it. It certainly isn't fun, but it's enormously productive and rewarding.

If you think that this is merely a matter of semantics, tell me—is childbirth fun? Is getting up in the middle of the night with a sick infant enjoyable? What if you read an article that said "child rearing has to be fun, or you won't stick with it"?

I want you to continue being turned on by strength training. To do so, however, you must recognize it for what it is—unpleasant, hard work. Do not try to enjoy it. Simply learn to endure it. Your rewards will be astronomical if you understand and apply these new ideas.

Fun—yes, you need it in your life. But first, get that extra fat off your body and continue to strengthen your major muscles. Soon you'll be able to get back involved with your aerobic classes. When you do, you'll do so knowing that you're leaner, stronger, and less prone to injury.

As a result, you'll have even more fun!

Better Business

Q. *I'm amazed at how much better my business associates treat me now that I've lost most of my fat. What's the connection here?*

A. You're right. Many of my ASAP participants have noted the same thing. Rightfully or wrongfully, a lean physique tells the world that discipline and motivation reside inside. True or not, it matters little because the perception might as well be the reality.

First impressions are certainly not everything, but a poor one sure takes a long time to overcome. No matter how smart, sincere, or wonderful you are, your appearance acts as a filter through which almost everything else is judged.

Physiology speaks even before you do. If anything the least bit articulate comes out of the mouth of a lean body, the intelligence is assessed in glowing terms.

Sadly, the same words spoken by someone who is overfat don't land with as much impact. The person doing the encountering would be skeptical: If this person's so sharp, why doesn't he do something to lose weight?

Your physical appearance can be an asset, or a liability, or maybe it's just neutral. You don't have to become obsessed with winning a bodybuilding contest. The right business suit is a great equalizer, so long as the body inside is within shooting distance of its ideal body-fat level.

As I've noted several times previously, getting a leaner, stronger body puts you in control of your own destiny. You should expect more good things to start happening to you in the future.

Strength in Age

Q. I remember that the average age of your ASAP participants was thirty-seven years. Who's the oldest person you've worked with?

A. That's an interesting question. If you examine all of the nineteen success stories that are featured in this book, you'll find that five of them are over fifty-nine. The oldest man was Phil Haisley, sixty-two, who lost 22¼ pounds of fat in six weeks. You can see Phil's before-and-after results on page 88.

Of the 109 women who were involved in the ASAP research, the oldest woman was Terry Mull at sixty-nine years of age. Terry, at a height of five feet three inches and a starting body weight of 149 pounds, did exceptionally well. Of the twenty-eight women in June of 1996 who started the course with Terry, over the first two weeks Terry did the best. She lost 8¼ pounds of fat and 1⅞ inches off her waist. Her muscle-building ability was indeed impressive. She added 3 pounds in only two weeks. Who says a sixty-nine-year-old woman can't build muscle?

I couldn't help but notice Terry during her first strength-training session. She was determined to master the wall squat and the negative push-up, which can be very challenging for most people. Within three workouts, she had the form down—which was especially motivating to the other women. Furthermore, Terry had never done any strength training in her life. She completed the six-week course with a fat loss of fourteen pounds.

"I'm really enjoying the way my slacks fit now," Terry said afterward. "And I got out a pair of shorts the other day from what seemed like a previous lifetime ago. My husband says I ought to start wearing them again. I believe I will."

Sometimes older people can get better results from strength training than younger people, noted Dr. William Evans and Dr. Irwin Rosenberg in their book, *Biomarkers: The 10 Determinants of Aging You Can Control*. The reason has to do with the significant amounts of muscle shrinkage, or atrophy, that many older people have. Such shrinkage responds very quickly to the right type of strength training. Drs. Evans and Rosenberg focused, in some of their studies, on training people in their nineties. They found that the positive muscle-building results were dramatic, even with this group.

So your age shouldn't be a significant factor in your getting involved with the ASAP program. Being older might even be an advantage for you. Of course, you'll still want to confer with your doctor beforehand.

Short Buddies

Q. Who's the shortest person who has been involved in the ASAP program?

A. In my introductory meetings, I always caution short people who join my course to realize some of the problems they must deal with. The primary problem centers around the lack of body surface area that a short person, compared to a tall person, has available to the environment for heat loss. This puts a short person at a disadvantage, especially when she's got several women in her group who are eight or nine inches taller.

In my September 1996 class of eighteen women, three of them were only five feet tall. Because Lydia Maree, the instructor I mentioned in chapter 7, is under five feet herself, she likes to get buddy-buddy with all the short women.

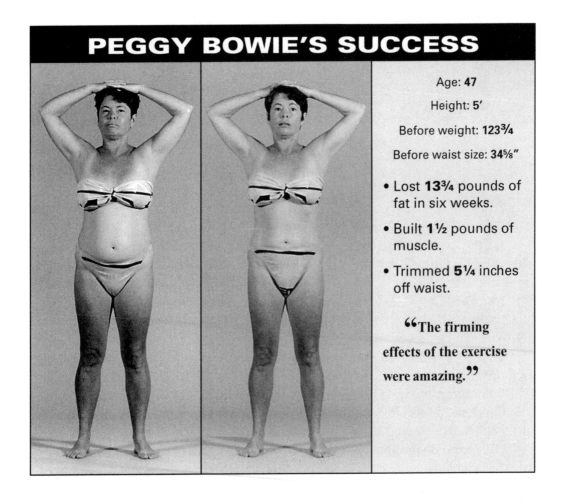

PEGGY BOWIE'S SUCCESS

Age: **47**

Height: **5'**

Before weight: **123¾**

Before waist size: **34⅝"**

- Lost **13¾** pounds of fat in six weeks.
- Built **1½** pounds of muscle.
- Trimmed **5¼** inches off waist.

"The firming effects of the exercise were amazing."

Well, I'm telling you, whatever she did worked like a charm. Rather than finish the course ranked near the bottom of the fat-loss listing, each of these women was very near the top. For example:

- Sonia Tergas, at five feet and fifty-two years of age, lost 16 pounds of fat and 4¾ inches off her waist.
- Beverly Hanks, at four feet eleven inches and fifty-nine years of age, lost 13¼ pounds of fat and 6⅜ inches off her waist.
- Peggy Bowie, at five feet and forty-seven years of age, lost 13¾ pounds of fat and 5¼ inches off her waist.

Actually, I've talked with Lydia several times since then, and I have a pretty good idea what she does with the short women. She encourages them to adhere to the rules with 100 percent compliance, with absolutely *no cheating*. Under those circumstances, the synergy works to the maximum degree. Thus, if you are shorter than normal and want to get results similar to your taller sisters, you've got to toe the line and stick to the rules.

Thank you, Lydia Maree, for your magic . . . and for your inspiring synergy. And I promise, one of my next projects will zero in on nothing but short women.

Champions at Losing Fat

Q. Of all the people you've worked with, who lost the most fat?
A. In 1996 alone, I've seen some dramatic fat losses.

Jeffrey Arnold, pictured on page 74, lost the most of the men: 33¾ pounds plus 20½ pounds, or a total of 54¼ pounds of fat from two courses or twelve weeks.

Tom Durkin lost the most from one six-week course: 37¼ pounds of fat.

Barrie Gaffney, pictured on page 22, lost the most of the women from one six-week course: 23½ pounds of fat.

Prior to 1996, some of the people who progressed through eighteen weeks or more were impressive.

Barry Ozer, pictured on page 180, lost 71¼ pounds of fat in eighteen weeks.

Carolyn Cannon lost the most of any women I've worked with: 47 pounds of fat in twenty weeks.

The grand champion of fat loss, however, is a man I worked with in 1993.

Larry Freedman, pictured on page 221, weighed in at 306 pounds. From his first program, he dropped 52¾ pounds of fat. I've never had anyone remove that much fat in six weeks. He continued with the course for three more six-week sessions.

At the end of six months, Larry's fat loss totaled 116½ pounds and 15½ inches off his waist.

Some of Larry's friends who hadn't seen him for six months didn't recognize him afterward. The change was so dramatic that a few of his friends didn't believe it was him—even after he told them who he was.

I haven't seen Larry in more than two years. Unfortunately, I've heard from reliable sources that he's regained about half of the fat he lost. If that's true, then Larry—as much as anyone I've worked with—understands what to do. It

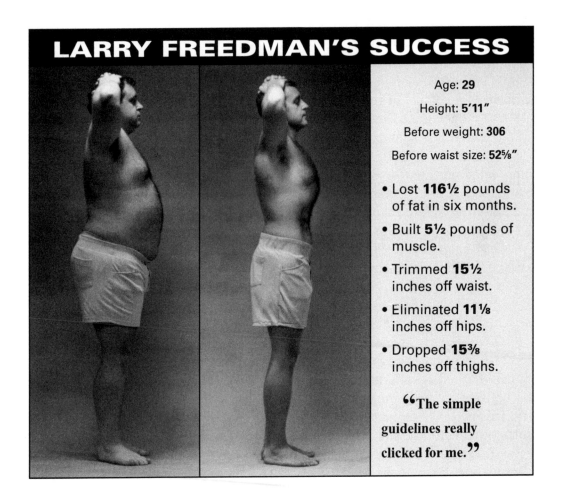

LARRY FREEDMAN'S SUCCESS

Age: **29**

Height: **5'11"**

Before weight: **306**

Before waist size: **52⅝"**

- Lost **116½** pounds of fat in six months.

- Built **5½** pounds of muscle.

- Trimmed **15½** inches off waist.

- Eliminated **11⅛** inches off hips.

- Dropped **15⅜** inches off thighs.

"The simple guidelines really clicked for me."

begins with those five words under Science: *Satiation, Strength, Superhydration, Sleep,* and *Synergy.*

He applied the necessary discipline once and he can do it again.

The First Two Weeks

Q. In your overall six-week averages for fat loss, men lose twenty-three pounds and women lose 15 pounds. I find it interesting that in the first two weeks men reduce eleven pounds and women reduce seven pounds. Why do men and women lose more during the first two weeks than during other two-week periods?

A. Yes, you're correct with your observation. Almost everyone who participates in my six-week course drops more fat during the first two-week period than during any other two-week time. As I pointed out in chapter 7, if you can communicate to your body that everything is all right, your system gives up its stored fat efficiently and quickly. But too much stress in even one area—such as lack of sleep, as Paige Arnold experienced—can prevent fat loss, or slow it significantly. The bottom line is to practice all the guidelines exactly as described. More of any of the recommendations is not better.

The longer you adhere to the guidelines, the more your body learns how to adapt. One way it adapts is to slow your metabolism. That's why building muscle, as you are losing fat, helps to curb this slowing. But since most people have more fat pounds to lose than they have muscle pounds to build, there is still an overall decrease in metabolism. That explains why your last five pounds is so much harder to lose than your first five pounds. You can thank, or detest, your Ice Age ancestors for this genetic trait.

Once again, knowledge and the understanding and application of it are the keys to getting your excessive fat off, finally and forever.

The Great Escape

Q. Everyone talks about losing fat. My question may sound dumb, but where does the fat go when you lose it?

A. Rather than dumb, it's actually intriguing. To answer this question, the fat within your body must be thought of in the context of physics and chemistry. This is the same physics and chemistry that apply throughout our known solar system. You should understand by now that fat translates to calories, and calories are units of heat energy. Heat emerges from your body in three ways—through your skin, lungs, and urine. Although you lose a small amount of heat through your feces, it is not thought to be significant unless you suffer from diarrhea.

Years ago, Albert Einstein and other scientists proved that you cannot create or destroy energy. You can only transfer it.

Thus, when you lose fat, what happens is you transfer heat energy out of your body into the environment. Once in the environment, it is available for use by other living organisms and by the environment. With each use, heat energy is once again transferred, and the cycle continues endlessly.

Transfer and More Transfer

Q. *So there's fat floating almost everywhere, right?*

A. Not exactly. But there is heat energy everywhere. The sun is our ultimate source of heat, and the key to understanding solar energy is the transfer concept.

Humans have no way to take in this energy directly. But plants can trap solar energy by using it to combine carbon dioxide and water. The product of this combination is a hydrated carbon, or carbohydrate. Only plants have the ability to grow by combining energy from the sun with the elements from the air, soil, and water. Animals usually get their energy from consuming plants. Humans get energy from eating both plants and animals.

In simple terms, the sun transfers heat to plants, and plants transfer heat to animals. Both plants (through carbohydrates) and animals (through proteins and fats) transfer heat to humans. Humans transfer heat back to the environment, plants, and other animals. Thus, all of these transfers have the capacity to change their forms (solid, liquid, and gas) and places of availability. It's an intriguing principle that needs to be publicized much more.

Skin Training

Q. *What can I do to make my skin more efficient at getting rid of heat calories?*

A. This is another provocative question that involves a fascinating answer. How efficient your skin is at eliminating calories depends on the blood flow through it. Your skin, as well as being your largest organ, it also very vascular. It is filled with arteries, capillaries, and veins. As you shrink your surface fat, the vessels in your skin will become more prevalent.

The main purpose of this large vascular supply is to enable your skin to function as a means of controlling the removal of calories and thereby govern your body temperature. Here is where proper strength training comes into the picture.

There is no better way to condition your skin than to strength train the underlying muscles. With proper strength training, you can isolate almost any part of your body—from the little muscles of your feet and hands to the large muscles of your thighs and chest—which pumps blood to those specific areas. This surging blood brings nutrients and heat. The rising heat in the muscle must then be released through your skin. And your skin learns to adapt better by becoming a more efficient heat regulator.

Lower-Back Pain and Trunk Curls

Q. My lower back hurts when I perform the trunk curl. Am I doing something wrong?

A. Yes, you're probably arching your lower back slightly during the start of the trunk curl. Here's what to do: Focus on keeping your lower back pressed against the floor. Do this as you begin curling your shoulders slowly off the floor. Once you get to the top position, focus again on pressing against the floor with your lower back as you smoothly return to the starting position. Use the same technique when you perform the trunk curl with twist.

Negative Push-Ups

Q. My lower back is fine during the trunk curl, but it hurts on the negative push-up. What should I do?

A. On the negative push-up, you're probably sagging your belly and hips—which arches your lower back—instead of keeping your torso, hips, and thighs perfectly straight. The negative push-up is properly performed by allowing your arms, but not your back, to bend. Viewed from the side, your torso lowers and your chest touches the floor before your hips and thighs. Be careful also not to jut your chin forward as you flex your elbows. Concentrate on bending your arms and leading with your chest.

Knee Problems and Wall Squats

Q. My knees are the problem, and they bother me on the wall squat. Should I continue doing it?

A. The wall squat is a great movement for your hips and thighs. Unfortunately, it can stress your knees. You may be unnecessarily impinging the joints, however, by having your heels too close to the wall. Make sure your heels are far enough away from the wall so that, when you are in the bottom position and viewed from the side, your calves are approximately parallel with the wall. Do not lean your torso or head forward. Focus intensely on contracting the large muscles of your thighs and hips.

Of the 109 women who progressed through the ASAP course, there wasn't a single one who didn't quickly adapt to the wall squat using the above instructions. Even those who had problem knees adjusted well. Work at it, and it will work for you.

Mysterious Bruising

Q. *I'm four weeks into the ASAP course, and I'm noticing some bruising on my thighs. Why?*

A. Don't fret. Such bruising is the result of an increased level of estrogen that circulates in the body of a woman who is losing fat. Somehow this weakens the capillaries and causes them to break under even the slightest pressure. When this happens, blood escapes and a bruise occurs.

Estrogen is broken down in your liver, and so is fat. When you are reducing, your liver preferentially breaks down the fat, leaving a greater-than-normal amount of estrogen in your bloodstream. Supplementing your eating with a hundred milligrams of vitamin C per day will help toughen the walls of the capillaries.

Cold Sensitivity

Q. *After losing fifteen pounds, I seem to be more sensitive to cold. Why?*

A. Some women who go through the ASAP course do complain about being cold some of the time. Even during the summer, air-conditioning can bring on the chills. So can superhydration.

Much of your fat is located right under your skin and acts as insulation. Once you thin this insulation, it's no wonder that you become more sensitive to cold. Your fingers, toes, and even the tip of your nose can be affected.

Before you put on a sweater or coat, remember that the state of almost shivering is one of the best ways to burn calories. Move around, take a walk, and try to keep that sweater off a little longer. You can train your body to generate its own heat. You'll burn more fat in the process.

Lower-Ab Work

Q. When I do the at-home exercises described in chapter 11, I feel it more in my upper abs. I need to work my lower abs. What can I do for them?

A. If you are doing the recommended exercises—trunk curl, trunk curl with twist, and reverse trunk curl—you *are* working your lower-abdominal muscles, but you will never feel the effect in the lower area as much as you do in the upper area. Here are the reasons why.

First, the largest section of your abdominal muscles is high on your waist, under your rib cage—not low or beneath your navel. You almost always feel abdominal exercises most in the mass of the muscles and toward the origin.

Second, the long, paired rectus abdominis muscles originate under your rib cage and insert into your pelvis. But when these muscles get near the region of your navel, they actually plunge through an opening in the horizontally crossing transverse abdominis muscles. The transverse abdominis, which lies on top of the insertion point of the rectus abdominis, tends to reduce the sensitivity of the deeper rectus abdominis.

Third, muscles begin their contractile process at the ends, where the tendons attach to the bones, and move gradually toward the center. Thus, to work the portion of the rectus abdominis that inserts on the pelvis, you have to move very slowly at the beginning of each exercise. Make sure you don't jerk quickly through the start of each exercise. Work diligently at mastering the super-slow protocol. If you can perform the reverse trunk curl very slowly, you should be able to generate additional feeling into the lower-abdominal area—especially as the involved muscles get stronger.

Fourth, sometimes bringing the iliopsoas muscles—which connect to your spine and thigh bones and lie underneath the abdominal muscles—into action can synergize feeling in the region below your navel. If you are strong enough, you may want to try the hanging leg raise, which is described on page 190.

Fifth, many people confuse working their lower abs with the removal of fatty deposits below their navel. Remember, working the lower abs does not draw calories from fat that may lie near the involved muscles. Spot reduction of fat is a myth.

Help for Love Handles

Q. My body fat seems to be thickest over my sides. Can I ever get rid of these love handles?

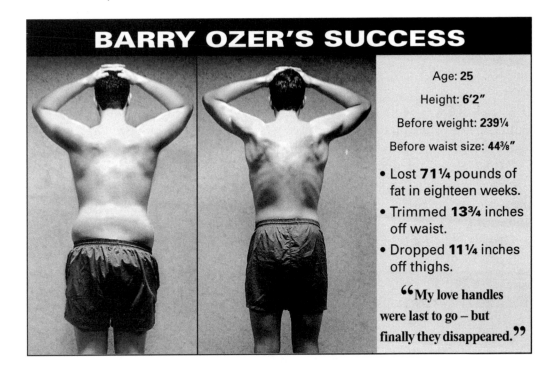

BARRY OZER'S SUCCESS

Age: **25**

Height: **6'2"**

Before weight: **239¼**

Before waist size: **44⅜"**

- Lost **71¼** pounds of fat in eighteen weeks.
- Trimmed **13¾** inches off waist.
- Dropped **11¼** inches off thighs.

"My love handles were last to go – but finally they disappeared."

A. I understand what you're talking about. Many men store fat first on the sides of their waist, which means that it will be the last to come off. *First on, last off* is one of the basic principles of fat deposition and reduction.

I want you to look at the above before-and-after photos of Barry Ozer. The time between the photos was eighteen weeks. Barry had some of the thickest love handles that I've ever seen. But they did not start shrinking significantly until the thirteenth week. By the end of the eighteenth week—and after a reduction of 13¾ inches from his waist—his love handles had shrunk to the point that they were unnoticeable.

So, yes, you can get rid of your love handles. Even if it takes you eighteen weeks, you can do it.

Sure you'll be challenged and tempted along the way. But you can combat each challenge and each temptation with discipline and patience.

You can conquer your love handles with *A Flat Stomach ASAP*.

Hip and Thigh Focus

Q. *Besides this fat around my stomach, I have considerable flab around my backside—especially my hips and thighs. Do I need to do anything special to focus on these areas?*

A. Since spot reduction of fat isn't possible, an overall program is best. You can't control your inherited patterns of where and to what degree you store and lose fat. Your best bet is to attack your problem areas with science.

Once again, I want you to examine some before-and-after photos. Look at the comparison of Barrie Gaffney below. Barrie lost most of her 23½ pounds of fat from her backside. Compare the differences in her buttocks, thighs, knees, and calves.

Did she do anything special in her strength-training routine? No.

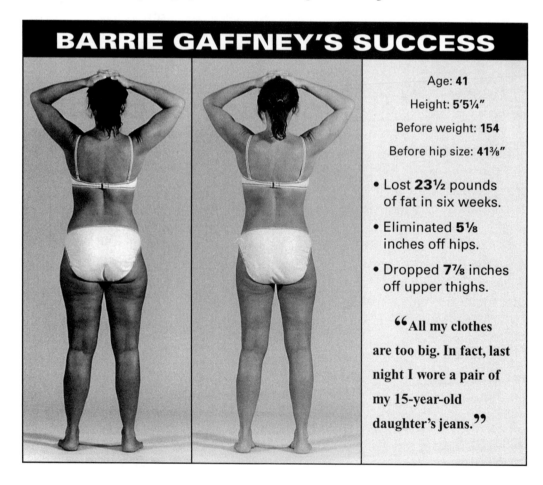

BARRIE GAFFNEY'S SUCCESS

Age: **41**

Height: **5'5¼"**

Before weight: **154**

Before hip size: **41⅜"**

- Lost **23½** pounds of fat in six weeks.

- Eliminated **5⅛** inches off hips.

- Dropped **7⅞** inches off upper thighs.

"All my clothes are too big. In fact, last night I wore a pair of my 15-year-old daughter's jeans."

Did she eat any unusual foods? No.

Did she supplement her program with aerobics on her off days? No.

What Barrie Gaffney did was to believe the ASAP program would work for her problems.

She did everything according to the book, with 100 percent compliance.

Do the same—and your results just may exceed your expectations.

The Best Solution

Q. *Are you saying that* A Flat Stomach ASAP *is a cure not only for a protruding belly and heavy hips and thighs, but also for problem areas throughout the body?*

A. No, the ASAP program is not a cure-all for what ails you. This action course and the principles that it is based on are the remedy for overfatness.

To determine the best solution to a problem requires the use of science. Science entails systematized knowledge derived from study and experimentation. For more than thirty years, I've studied and experimented with various eating and exercising plans to help people lose fat and build muscle.

While there are many different books and plans that claim to provide solutions to the problem of being overfat in the United States, I believe the one I'm sharing with you in this book is the most effective and efficient. The proof of the program is in the results, and I challenge any other program to come forth with its data and before-and-after pictures.

I first presented this challenge to a national fitness convention in 1985, after I showed a dozen slides of people who have been through a ten-week diet and exercise plan. I've repeated the same challenge many times since then. A few people have been upset and have argued aggressively with me concerning their methods and practices, but no one has ever produced data and before-and-after photographs that were equal to, or more impressive, than mine.

I'm also a realist. My approach is *not* for everyone. In fact, during my introductory meetings I always turn off a few people with my disciplined rules. Therefore, they don't get involved. Even among those who do join, some people drop out and some get only marginal benefits.

But most people who stick with the guidelines see results: measurable results after only two weeks, and dramatic results—the kinds you can observe from a quick glance at before-and-after pictures—in six weeks. If they continue for another four to six weeks, their lives just may change completely.

And you don't have to take my word for it. Thumb back through this book and reexamine the success stories.

These stories are about real people, whose names have *not* been changed, who freely allowed me to use their photographs, measurements, and interviews.

These are real people—just like you and your neighbors—who have jobs, spouses, kids, pains and problems, and highs and lows—just like you do.

If you've been through the ASAP program, then you know what I'm talking about. You've already taken the necessary steps and you've progressed through six weeks. You've experienced the great results. But you must continue with more of the same—and you will.

If you haven't started the ASAP course yet, then it's time that you did.

Simply, it takes *motivation* and *know-how.* You already have the motivation, or you wouldn't have made it this far in the book. This course provides you with specific know-how. And that know-how centers around

Awareness

Science

Application

Persistence

It's time for *your* flat stomach and *your* lean body to emerge—ASAP!

A special letter from Ellington Darden . . .

HOW TO GET EVEN BETTER RESULTS FASTER!

Dear Reader,

I want to share with you some cutting-edge research that became finalized in my mind only weeks before the publication of this book.

If you take full advantage of my discovery, and combine it with the listed guidelines in this ASAP course, then I firmly believe that you'll achieve even *better results faster.*

In the last chapter of this manual, on page 212, I mentioned the concept of *metabolic equilibrium.* Metabolic equilibrium means keeping your body's energy production stable.

When you're in metabolic equilibrium, your body feels protected. None of your bio-defense mechanisms are triggered. You're able to concentrate better on specific goals. Therefore, your body can lose fat and build muscle more efficiently and more effectively.

Metabolic equilibrium is governed primarily by your blood glucose.

When you wake up in the morning, your blood probably contains between 70 and 100 milligrams of glucose in each 100 milliliters of blood. This range, which is known as the fasting blood glucose concentration, is normal and is accompanied by a feeling of alertness and well-being.

If you don't eat, your blood glucose level gradually falls. At 65 to 60 milligrams per 100 milliliters, slightly below the normal range, you'll feel hungry and be motivated to eat. Eating will bring your glucose back into the normal range.

It's important, however, that the blood glucose level not rise too high. A meal too high in calories or too high in certain nutrients, for example, can excessively elevate your glucose levels. Doing so sets off a chain reaction that causes you to become very efficient at storing fat. Obviously, this is not what you want—especially if you are trying to reduce.

Nothing—and I mean literally *nothing* that I've tried in more than thirty years of working with overfat people—has ever produced metabolic equilibrium like my new Perfect Score food supplement.

Tests that monitor blood glucose levels show that Perfect Score does a superior job of equalizing blood sugar. Perfect Score, served as a meal or a snack, stabilizes and maintains glucose levels between 70 and 85 milligrams per 100 milliliters of blood for two to three hours.

This rather narrow range appears to be ideal for the entire process of losing fat and building muscle. Furthermore, this range keeps you on an even keel with no hunger.

Perfect Score takes the complexities out of dieting. All you do is simply tear open a packet, mix the contents with cold water, and drink it down. In combination with the targeted ASAP eating and exercising, Perfect Score will help you achieve and maintain the look you've always wanted.

You have my personal guarantee: If Perfect Score isn't the best meal replacement, or metabolic equalizer, you've ever tried, then I'll refund every penny of your purchase price—no questions asked.

I'm betting, however, that you'll be not only satisfied, but elated.

That's why if you're serious—*really serious*—about losing fat, building muscle, and flattening your stomach in the fastest possible way . . . then I'd like you to pick up the phone and call toll-free: 1-888-256-2727.

If you qualify, I'd like you to participate in a unique Perfect Score ASAP plan. A limited supply of Perfect Score will be available at a special discount. But you must hurry while the supply lasts.

Remember, this project is for serious women and men only.

Yes, you can lose fat and flatten your stomach in record time. And the key is to maintain metabolic equilibrium.

Sincerely,

Ellington Darden

P.S. If you order now, I'll send you my 37-minute videotape, which illustrates the complete *A Flat Stomach ASAP* course. This $19.95 videotape shows you how to perform all the recommended exercises in perfect form. And it's yours FREE!

Call toll-free: 1-888-256-2727